# FIT IN THE MIDDLE
## Your Belly May Be Telling You Something

A Journey through Metabolic Syndrome
Health and Nutrition

by

Gregg Ghelfi

Cover Design by Cynthia Morrison

Illustrations by Rick Menard
www.rickmenard.com

Dedicated to Cyndi and Emily

# CONTENTS

# ACKNOWLEDGMENTS

I would like to thank a number of people whom have helped contribute to this book. Bob Ghelfi and Marilee Tatom were instrumental in providing direction, offering medical, nutritional and fitness advice and making sure the substance of this book was realistic and valid. I would like to thank Brent and Jan Ghelfi for taking the time to read and critique early drafts; Paul Thayer for his editing; Laurie Harper for her advice; and Tim Dwyer for his inspiration. Finally I would like to thank my wife, Cyndi, for her comments and putting the book into its final form.

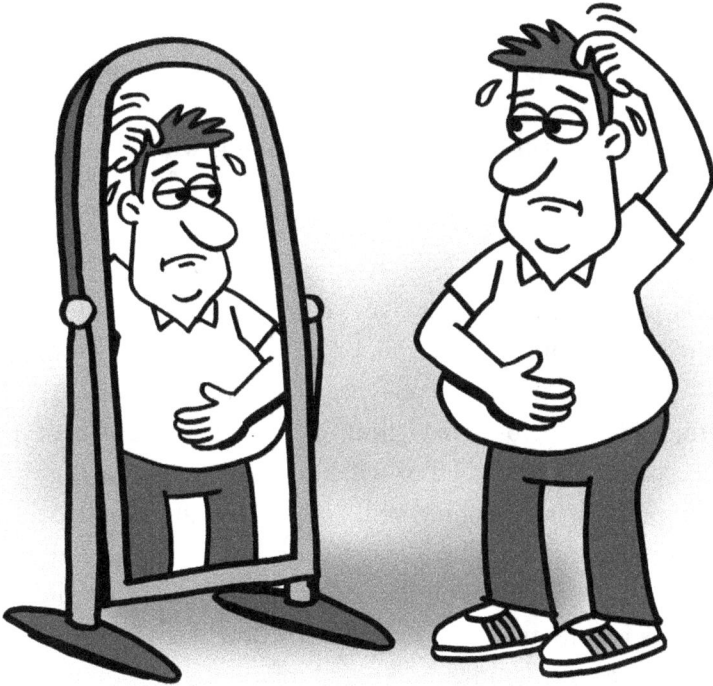

# 1

## HOW DID I GET HERE?

Steve stared into the mirror. He hardly recognized the person in it. At five feet, ten inches and 235 pounds, he was a bloated version of himself. His face was round, and his chin and neck had become one. His once well-defined chest was a roll of flesh with a crease that ran from just under his nipples to below his armpits.

And look at that gut! Seven-month pregnant women had nothing on him. It was his most defining feature. You could almost rest a drink on it and, unless he leaned forward, it was the last part of his body he saw if he looked down. He rarely looked into the mirror anymore because he didn't like what he saw. And he never stepped on a scale.

But this week he had been forced to face his weight. Under a new company policy, he was required to get a complete physical. At forty-four, smack in the middle of life, he had undergone a variety of the kind of tests that all men dread, along with giving blood. The blood tests caused him the most concern. The doctor reviewed the results with him and noted a variety of numbers that were either above or below the recommended norm. She finished by telling him that the results indicated Metabolic Syndrome. He didn't know exactly what this was, but it didn't sound good.

"How did I get here?" he asked himself, still looking into the mirror. He had not always been overweight. He had been active in high school as a football and baseball player when he was 170 pounds and in peak physical condition. And he remained in shape through his twenties. As an electrician, he wired houses and office buildings, which was physically demanding work that required him to be in hot buildings pulling wires through framed houses and setting up electrical panels. On weekends, he played on various club sports' leagues, including basketball and softball teams. At his ten-year reunion he had looked as good if not better than he did when he graduated from high school.

The year of his tenth reunion was also the year of another milestone. His wife, Beth, was pregnant with their first child. He had met Beth on a blind date four years before. She was five years his senior, and she had a daughter, Ronda, from a previous marriage.

He soon learned that parenthood brought great joy and major changes. He began substituting participation in sports for coaching sports. His time after work was booked with parenting rather than exercising.

His job also changed. He went from being an electrician to being an estimator. Instead of toiling in a hot building he worked at a computer. Aside from the gardening, he hired a lawn service to do the yard work. His favorite pastime was boating at the lake, but the weather in Seattle limited his boating time to a couple of months in the summer. Aside from sports, he was not much of a television watcher, but he liked doing role-playing video games on his computer. He also spent a lot of time going to games and practices with his son, Zack, now fifteen, and his daughter, Sara, now ten.

Steve either skipped breakfast or he grabbed a soft drink and a donut or a candy bar or muffin at the convenience store on his way to work. Lunch consisted of either fast food or a quick meal at a sit-down restaurant, where he liked to eat a chicken salad sandwich and a soda. He usually snacked on chips or a candy bar around three because he felt tired and needed sugar to keep him going to the end of the day. In the evening he drank a beer and joined the family for either a sit-down meal of chicken or fish and potatoes or corn or boxed or frozen food that was quick and easy to prepare.

Beth was a forty-nine-year-old proud mother of three children. Her twenty-three year-old daughter, Ronda, had recently graduated from college. Beth hadn't participated in high school athletics, but she was a runner in college. She had her daughter the year she graduated from college, and despite starting a career as an accountant and raising a child, she managed to run three to five miles a day, five days a week.

That changed after she married Steve and she had Zack. Her weight increased from 120 to 165 pounds during the pregnancy. While she was able to lose her pregnancy weight within six months after having Ronda, she couldn't get below 130 pounds after Zack. Then, after she had Sara, she couldn't - get below 140 pounds. She was busy with her job, and while she had dual custody with her ex-husband in raising Ronda, she had her hands full raising Zack and Sara.

At five feet four inches and 145 pounds, she was in the high normal range of weight. She was too busy to run, and she had never participated in weight training or team sports. Her job as a chief financial officer at a nursing home kept her at her desk or in meetings. She enjoyed working on her garden on the weekends and walking her dog.

She didn't feel as if she ate too much. She had coffee with cream and sugar along with a bagel or muffin in the morning. She normally took her lunch to work. She liked chicken salad sandwiches, potato chips, and diet colas. Because she worked in a large office, there was always a cake or donuts to celebrate a birthday or anniversary. In the evening she might have a glass of wine, but usually she just drank lemonade or water. She had smoked in high school but had stopped after becoming pregnant and had never taken it up again.

Steve and Beth were looking forward to the upcoming weekend, when they would fly to Phoenix for Steve's twenty-five year high school reunion. It was November now, when Seattle was cold and cloudy, but the weather in Phoenix would be great. Steve had left Phoenix twenty years before, and his family had moved a few years after that, but he returned when he could to reminisce with old friends. He had been to the tenth and twentieth reunions. For Steve, reunions were a reminder of simpler days gone by. Beth looked forward to the resort, the spa, and the pool. She had become friends with a few of the classmates and their spouses, but high school wasn't the greatest time for her, and Steve always overindulged and reverted to the ways of an idiotic teenager.

But the test results from his physical put a damper on the trip. The doctor had mentioned a number of medications she could prescribe but advised him that his best bet was to lose weight, especially in his belly. He had talked to Beth about the appointment and the doctor's suggestions the night before. Neither of them had ever been on a diet, and while they had seen infomercials on miracle weight-loss diets, they had not paid any attention to what they ate or their activities. He was not a fan of taking medications, so losing weight seemed like the best option. But how?

He preferred not to think about it this weekend. Vacations were a time to have fun and not worry about things. But the doctor had talked about long-term heart issues. That got his attention. His uncle had died at the age of fifty-five, leaving two teenage daughters fatherless. He didn't know if the heart attack was preventable, but he knew how it affected his cousins. He was determined not to leave his children too early because of something he could prevent.

When he packed his bag, he put his blood test records in his carryon bag. He knew that one of his former classmates was a doctor. Maybe she could explain the results to him. Maybe they weren't all bad and his doctor was being overly cautious. In any event, the doctor had talked to him about excess calories, decreased metabolism, and a lack of exercise. He had understood about twenty-five percent of what she said. He had tried to explain it to Beth, but she was just as much in the dark as he was. Perhaps someone at the reunion could explain in English what it all meant.

"I left plenty of food in the refrigerator and the number for the resort on the counter next to the phone," Beth said to Ronda, who had agreed to watch Zack and Sara for the weekend. "And you have our cell numbers."

"I'm twenty-three years old, Mom," Ronda said. "I think I can handle it for the two days you're gone."

"Yeah, Mom," said Zack, interrupting his video game long enough to join in "I'll take care of things."

Beth just stared at Zack and nodded at Ronda. She still saw her children as toddlers. "Yes, yes, I'm just making sure."

Steve hugged Ronda and Sara and shook Zack's hand. Sara looked genuinely sad to see them leave. Zack looked as if he was already planning a party as he smiled and hugged Beth.

"Don't do anything I wouldn't do, Zack," Steve said. He briefly flashed back to his younger days and hoped that Zack wouldn't do any of the things he had done.

"I won't, Dad," Zack said. 'Aside from work, play games, watch sports and eat, what does my dad do?' he wondered.

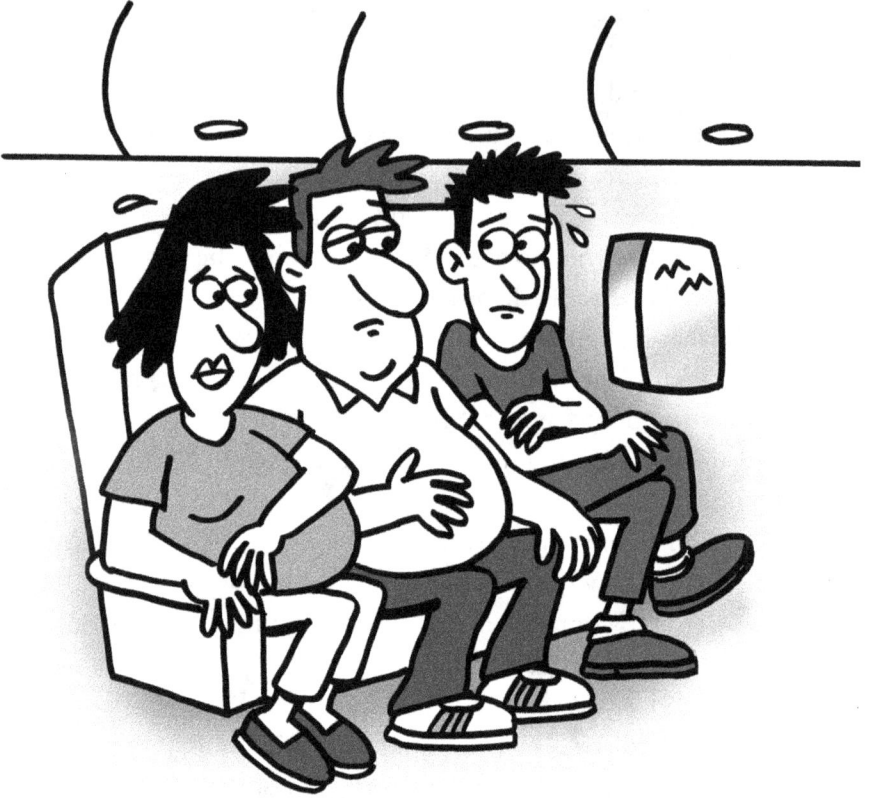

# 2

## WHAT IS METABOLIC SYNDROME?

Airports are great people-watching places, Steve thought. Older men and women anxiously awaited the metal detectors, where menacing eyes searched their bags and those with an artificial hip volunteered themselves to be probed and prodded like prisoners back from the quarry. Children clanked their toys, whined at their parents, and tumbled down the aisles. Buddies met at the bar to start their weekend of poker or golf. Boyfriends anticipated a weekend with their girlfriend, and girlfriends rejoiced as their boyfriends left. Professional travelers glared at them all.

Steve and Beth did not categorize them in that way. What they saw was a lot of overweight people. "Why was the doctor saying that I had to lose weight?" Steve asked. "Look at all the fat people."

What he saw was not an anomaly.

Every few years the Center for Disease Control and Prevention conducts a survey focusing on health topics.[1] It is not a pretty picture. Three out of four men are either overweight or obese.[2] One out of three men is obese. Not to be outdone, two out of three women are overweight or obese, and more than one out of three is obese. The percentage of obese men and women has more than doubled since the early 1970s. Even children are getting in on the act. The number of obese children has more than tripled, and obesity in young children ages two to five has increased by over 40 percent since they started surveying for children that young.[3]

Steve and Beth were a little early. "You want to grab a drink to start our vacation?" Steve asked.

"Sure, I could use a Margarita to get into the spirit of the southwest."

They sidled up to the bar and ordered a Margarita for Beth and an Alaskan Amber for Steve.

"Here's to a great weekend," said Steve, lifting his glass. He eyed her and then looked up at the television.

She sighed, assuming that he meant a great weekend of drinking, eating, and relaxing. He couldn't be referring to a great physical weekend. His sex drive had diminished along with his energy over the past ten years, and she had lost a lot of her sex drive over the past few years. They still had sex, but it was more and more rare.

But Steve's thinking had moved past the toast. He stared at the television, watching an infomercial about a fast and easy weight-loss diet. Everywhere you looked, it seemed, someone was talking about the insatiable appetites and rotund bodies of Americans. First Lady Michelle Obama had launched a campaign, "Let's Move," aimed at ending childhood obesity in one generation. Various reality television shows were dedicated to showing obese people losing weight, with great accolades and money to the winners. Every infomercial on weight loss or exercise claimed to help you lose weight with little or no effort. Stroll through the grocery store and peruse the labels: low fat, no trans fat, low calorie, no calorie, speed up your metabolism, gluten-free, vegan, high in protein, low in sugar, comes with a tapeworm.

"Maybe I'll try that diet," Steve said, pointing to the television, interrupting Beth's train of thought.

"Oh, Steve! You aren't going to start eating tofu are you?"

"I don't know what I'm gonna do. I just know that the doctor said that I need to make some changes or else I was in for a rude awakening sooner or later."

Silence met his words.

It was time to board. They had assigned seats but had elected to carry on their bags to save the baggage fee. Of course that meant hoping you weren't the last to board and finding you had a bag with no home.

Luckily, they were in the middle of the pack. They obediently trudged down the jet way to the plane like cattle heading to slaughter. They had aisle and middle seats. Steve drew the short straw and sat in the middle. Airplane seats are a cruel joke, he thought, for the big and tall. They stared at their seats, which looked as if they had been designed for toddlers. If you're much wider than a supermodel, your body crowds your neighbor's seat. If you're tall, your knees jam into the seatback in front of you. And that's before the seat reclines.

Beth and Steve wedged themselves into their seats, hoping no one was assigned the window seat.

But today was not their lucky day. A man with brown, spiky hair, about five-ten, with a build so slender he almost looked emaciated, tapped Beth on her shoulder and pointed to the window seat. He looked reluctantly at his accommodations for the next three hours as if he were the sardine that got stuck at the bottom of the can. Steve breathed a sigh of relief. At least they wouldn't be battling for the armrest.

The flight attendants predictably prattled on about being there for the passengers' safety. Steve had travelled enough to tune it out. He reached into his pocket and took out the papers with his lab work and other test results from his doctor and stared at them. It was all just as meaningless as before.

"Is that a report from your cardiologist?" asked the thin man next to him.

Steve involuntarily lowered the report and scowled.

"I'm sorry, I didn't mean to pry. My name is Paul. I'm a cardiologist from Tacoma. I just recognized the report."

Steve looked at him and said, "Hi, Paul, I'm Steve." Should he discuss the report with this stranger? On the one hand, his physical life in tests sat here, and according to his doctor, the picture was not pretty. On the other hand, this doctor may be able to explain the numbers, and maybe they aren't all that bad. "Yes, the report is from my cardiologist. I met with her on Thursday, and she didn't make it sound very good."

"I'm sorry to hear that," Paul replied.

"Maybe you can explain some of the numbers to me," Steve said, beginning to get excited. Maybe this doctor could explain the results to me in plain English. Perhaps he will tell me that it isn't all that bad.

"I would be happy to look at your lab results and explain them as best I can. Of course I'm not your doctor and would not be diagnosing you."

Steve handed Paul the report and turned to Beth and said, "Beth, if I drop dead on this flight, shoot the doc."

Paul gave him a half-hearted laugh, but he really wanted to ask Steve why heavy people always wear a Hawaiian shirt. He stopped himself and looked at the report.

After what seemed like an eternity to Steve, Paul put down the papers and looked at him. "Steve, I won't lie to you. The report isn't necessarily dire, but without some changes it could be. The results point to what is known as Metabolic Syndrome."

"My doctor said the same thing. What is that?"

"Metabolic Syndrome, or Syndrome X, has a number of definitions.   It's used to describe a cluster of symptoms that include insulin resistance, dyslipidemia, hypertension, and abdominal obesity.[4] A person with Metabolic Syndrome is on the short list for diabetes, cardiovascular disease, coronary heart disease, or stroke."

"That doesn't sound good," Steve said, his eyes wide.

"No, it isn't," Paul replied.   "In fact, in a study called the Helsinki Police Project, researchers followed 970 men over a twenty-two year period.   The men, average age forty-eight, were free of heart disease and diabetes at the beginning of the study.   A study done on the men who developed heart disease or stroke over the twenty-two-year period showed a direct link between heart disease and stroke and Metabolic Syndrome.   The results also indicated that insulin-resistance itself may enhance the development of atherosclerosis, the thickening of blood vessels.[5]"

"I'm forty-four, just four years younger than those guys in the study!   You got that information from my report?" Steve asked incredulously.   "What the hell are these symptoms, and how do you know I have them?"

"Steve, are you okay?" Beth asked.   She had nodded off, but Steve's raised voice had awakened her.

"Yes, perhaps this is not the appropriate place to discuss this," Paul suggested.   He stared at the dandruffed hair of the person in front of him, who was reclining almost into his lap.   He reflexively scratched his own scalp.

"I'm okay, Beth.   Sorry, Paul.   I would like you to continue."

"Perhaps it would make more sense if we went over your symptoms one at a time," Paul said.

Steve nodded.

"Let's start with insulin resistance because it's at the heart of Metabolic Syndrome," Paul began.   "Perhaps it's easiest to explain insulin resistance by starting with the food you eat.   You eat a piece of bread.   Your digestive system breaks down the bread into small parts that are able to seep through your intestines into your bloodstream.   One of these small parts is glucose.   Glucose is used to produce energy in our muscles and brain. But to be useful as energy, glucose must enter your cells from your bloodstream. Insulin escorts the glucose and acts like a key to the cells. If your muscles and brain have sufficient amounts of glucose, insulin puts the excess in the liver. If your liver is full, insulin stores glucose in fat cells.

"Unless you're a type one diabetic[6], insulin and glucose are great pals. You eat another piece of bread, the glucose comes through the intestines to the bloodstream, and insulin is there to escort it to the waiting cells. It's a simple and effective system unless you abuse it.

"But most people take unfair advantage of the system by eating or drinking too many simple carbohydrates in the form of bread, pizza, ice cream, cookies, and soft drinks. These foods and drinks may be okay once in a while, but many people ingest them every day for two or three meals a day. Unfortunately, your cells tire of this routine. They change the lock, and your insulin no longer has the key. The excess glucose has nowhere to go, so it roams your bloodstream wreaking havoc. Initially, we may become insulin-resistant, but over time you can get type two diabetes."

"Am I insulin-resistant?" Steve asked. "What in my results tells you this?"

Paul said, "Insulin resistance is tested by measuring the amount of glucose in the bloodstream after fasting. If the amount of glucose is 100 to 125 milligrams per deciliter, you are considered pre-diabetic. Once your fasting glucose goes over 125, you are considered diabetic. Your doctor will place you on medications designed to control the level of glucose. You may also need shots to control it. Your test results show that your blood glucose level was at one hundred and twelve. You aren't diabetic yet, but you're on your way.

"Insulin resistance and type two diabetes play major roles in cardiovascular disease, strokes, kidney disease, and nerve and retinal damage.[7]"

Steve stared past Paul, looking through the window at the endless, clear blue sky. His older brother had developed diabetes and failed to  do anything about it. He vividly remembered seeing his brother in the hospital after he had his right foot amputated.

"It also shows that you suffer from hypertension," Paul continued. "Hypertension is chronically elevated blood pressure. and you have hypertension when either the upper number is over 140 or the lower number is over 90. Your blood pressure was 142 over 88." [8]

"What causes high blood pressure?" Steve asked.

"There are a number of possible causes of high blood pressure. Excess fat cells attach themselves to blood vessels, thus decreasing the vessel diameter. Or chronic inflammation of your blood vessels can cause permanent damage to them. In either case pressure builds as blood vessels thicken and the inner diameter decreases. As the blood pressure builds, your body builds more muscles to aid in blood flow. The extra muscle decreases the pliability of the vessel, and a vicious cycle ensues.

"Hypertension is an indicator that your heart is working too hard. If it is not treated, it can lead to – you guessed it – heart failure."

"You're really making me feel great as I head to my class reunion, doc," Steve said. He was trying to concentrate, but the jerk behind him was using his tray table as a drum.

Steve ordered his second beer from the flight attendant. "We might as well continue," he said. "What is dyslipidemia?" Beth pretended to read a book while she listened to Paul.

"Dyslipidemia is an elevation of lipids, or fat cells, in the blood. The two forms of fat cells that are measured are cholesterol and triglycerides."

"I've had my cholesterol tested," Beth said. "It was around 170. I think I remember that being good."

"Yes, a lot of people are familiar with cholesterol," Paul replied, "and they know that a number below 200 is good and above 200 is bad. But there is more to cholesterol than a simple good or bad result. Cholesterol is a combination of fat, or lipids, and steroids. We use cholesterol to form cell membranes and other tissue and some hormones. The liver produces about eighty percent of our cholesterol, and the rest we get from our diet. Cholesterol comes in two major forms, High-Density Lipoprotein, or HDL, and Low-Density Lipoprotein, or LDL. HDL is actually good cholesterol."

"We have good cholesterol?" Steve said. "I didn't know that."

"Yes, we do, Steve," Paul replied. "HDL cholesterol helps remove LDL cholesterol, the bad cholesterol, and triglycerides from our bloodstream. When you were tested, they determined your HDL levels separately from your overall levels. A score of less than 40 in men and 50 in women indicates a risk factor for heart disease. A number over 60 is optimal for both men and women."

The flight attendant returned with Steve's beer.

"Low-Density Lipoprotein is the bad cholesterol," Paul continued, "because it forms plaque in our arteries.[9] The plaque decreases the diameter of our arteries and increases the risk of inflammation. Inflammation is our immune system's response to a perceived foreigner it wants out of our body. The immune cells congregate at the inflamed site and decrease the diameter of the blood vessel. When measuring LDL, less than a hundred is optimal, above one hundred twenty-nine is above optimal, and above a hundred and sixty is high."

"The total number is a combination of HDL and LDL," Paul explained. "This is where the infamous number 200 comes from, Beth. A number less than 200 is considered healthy; 200 to 240is borderline high; and a number over 240 is considered high, with an increase in the risk of coronary heart disease."

"So my 170 may not be good?" Beth asked.

"No, 170 is a good number," Paul said. "But were you at risk for coronary heart disease, the doctor would have done other tests, and your HDL levels would have been relevant.

"The other form of fat that was tested was your triglycerides,"[10] Paul continued. "Triglyceride levels are tested by measuring the amount that is roaming our blood vessels. Less than 100 milligrams per deciliter is optimal, one hundred to 190 is borderline high, 200 to 249 is high, and above 490 is very high. At the risk of repeating myself, an elevated blood count indicates an increased risk of cardiovascular disease and stroke."

Steve looked as if he had been punched in the gut. Beth leaned back in her chair. She hadn't taken the test results too seriously.

Doctors always cover their butts and paint worst-case scenarios, she thought. But this guy wasn't Steve's doctor. He was just some doctor sitting next to them on a plane.

"Are you saying that Steve is going to die soon?" Beth asked, looking alarmed.

"No, I'm not saying that," Paul replied. "I'm saying that his test results point to a person at risk for heart disease. And there is one other factor that the blood tests do not reveal but is nonetheless an important contributor to Metabolic Syndrome."

"What's that?" Beth said.

Steve remained silent, glumly staring at his glass of beer.

"Excess weight, specifically fat found around the stomach, is a factor in Metabolic Syndrome. The fat cells in your abdomen, called visceral fat, tend to be larger than other fat cells and more prone to rupture due to their size and the pressure variations that exist in the abdomen. These cell ruptures cause the immune system to kick in, causing inflammation.[11] This causes your arteries to clog and may lead to a heart attack or stroke."

Steve looked at his bulging stomach. He thought about punching Paul but decided that wouldn't be prudent.

Paul said, "Obesity is defined by the National Institute of Health as a BMI, or Body Mass Index, above thirty.[12] The BMI is a key index for relating body weight to height. You are overweight if your BMI is above twenty-five.

"If your weight and height in this report are accurate," Paul said as he used the calculator on his phone, "your body mass index is thirty-three. That is obese, according to the scale. Body Mass Index is a rough estimation of your body fat in relation to your total weight."

Steve didn't say anything. He knew he was fat but had never thought of himself as obese.

"That's a load of crap," Steve said. "I have friends who are muscular, and they would be considered overweight on that scale."

"I agree, it's not the best test, but it's an easy one for the government to use as a general guideline." If you want a better estimate, one of the simplest and most effective tests you can do is to measure your waist and determine your waist-to-hip ratio. A waist measurement, measured just above your navel, of greater than forty inches for men and thirty-five inches for women is considered high and one of the indicators of Metabolic Syndrome. And a waist-to-hip ratio of one or greater in men and point eighty-seven or greater in women of your age, Beth, is considered very high.

"Of course there are other ways to measure your actual body fat percentage, such as using skinfold calipers and hydrostatic weighing," [13] Paul said. "They are objective measurements that track your body's progress if done consistently each time. But for your purposes, your body weight, waist circumference, and your waist-to-hip ratio will do as measurements you can watch to measure your progress if you choose to lose weight."

Steve stared at his empty beer glass. He recalled joking with his buddies and even his children about how he worked hard at growing his "beer belly." To tell the truth, he wasn't happy about his gut, but after a while he had gotten used to it. Now his doctor and this jerk were telling him that his weight was killing him.

"Heart attacks, strokes!" Steve exclaimed, glaring at Paul. "What the heck! Because I'm a little overweight, you're telling me I'm on a short list to the ER."

Paul sighed, wishing he were sitting next to the crying baby a few rows back. "As I just said you can be overweight and not have Metabolic Syndrome. But weight is a factor in Metabolic Syndrome, and it's one you can control. A drop in weight should result in lower blood pressure, lower incidence of insulin resistance, and a decrease in cholesterol and triglycerides. In my practice, when a person comes in with body fat consolidated around the stomach, nine times out of ten he or she shows risks for heart disease in the blood work and physical.

"However, you can be overweight and perfectly satisfied with your body and your ability to move around. Thin people are not necessarily happier people. From a health standpoint, being slightly overweight is better for you than being too underweight.

"But even if you're one of the lucky few who don't have an increased risk of heart disease with excessive weight, you have a number of reasons to reduce it. "You are at a higher risk for cancer, arthritis, and gout. You are more likely to have breathing problems and difficulty sleeping. Travel is more difficult. Clothes do not fit properly. You are more apt to have ankle, knee, and hip problems. In short, overweight people have shorter and more uncomfortable lives than fit people do."

Paul sneaked a look at his watch. There was an hour left on the flight. Einstein didn't have to convince this group that time is relative. He was heading to Phoenix for a medical seminar and some golf. He enjoyed flying because it gave him time to relax; but this was painful.

Steve stared at his tray table.

Beth thought about herself. She was heavier than she used to be, but she didn't think she was overweight. However, her knees and back ached all the time. She was also tired and even felt depressed sometimes. She considered asking this doctor about her conditions, but she decided to remain silent.

Thirty minutes crawled by before she said, "Well, Doctor Doom, the man who looks as if he could eat a horse and not gain a pound, do you have any advice for your fat seatmates?"

Paul wished he had never started this conversation. He had spent his whole career delivering bad news or advice that went unheeded. He was used to hearing excuses about why a patient couldn't change even when not changing might result in disaster.

"First, you've just been hit with bad news," Paul said. "It's understandable that you're angry and confused. Two days ago, your lives were headed in a certain direction, and now they have unexpectedly changed course. My advice is to learn all you can about eating better and exercising. Even this weekend, ask your friends about exercise and food. Your doctor can prescribe lots of medications that will lower your cholesterol and your blood pressure. But medications have side effects, and they could mask your problems rather than cure them. You can go on a hard-core diet that would help you drop weight fast. But unless you made real changes, the weight will come back as fast as you lose it.

"Second, I wasn't always thin. Twelve years ago I weighed fifty more pounds than I do today. On a whim I decided to run around my block. It was less than a mile, but I was so out of shape I had to stop a couple of times, and I walked most of it. I was so disgusted with myself that I vowed to continue running and never allow myself to be in such lousy shape.

"As I exercised, I changed my diet. Within a year, I ran my first half marathon. Since that fateful day, I've run several marathons, including the Boston marathon three times. Running worked for me. Do your own research. Ask questions. Find physical activities that you enjoy. Find healthy foods that you can substitute for the unhealthy foods you currently like."

"Physical activity, healthy foods?" Steve said. "How do I know what foods are healthy or what type of exercises I should do? And how do I know it will do any good?"

The plane landed, and the passengers shoved their way toward the exit.

"Keep asking questions," Paul said. "You will find that the relationship between eating, exercise, and health to be very strong. With perseverance you will discover foods and exercise that you can enjoy for what will hopefully be a long and healthy life.

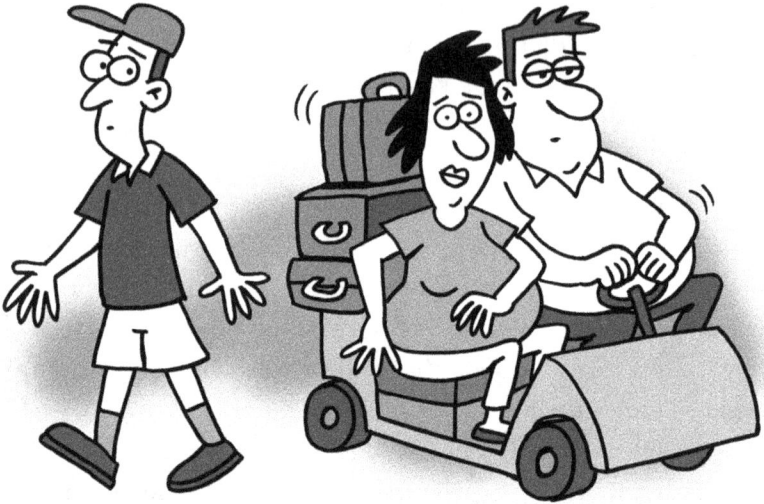

# 3

## NEAT

Steve and Beth hopped into a taxi and headed to the resort. The ride took about twenty-five minutes, so they had time to think. They had both been physically fit well into their twenties. Now they had gained thirty to sixty pounds, and they became tired during a walk around the neighborhood. Beth's knees and back hurt by the end of each day. Steve was looking at potential heart trouble as well as back pain. How had it come to this?

That was a good question. The National Health and Nutrition Examination Survey has shed light on the answer. Over the past forty years, caloric intake has gone up by slightly more than 200 calories for men. In the 1971-74 survey, men consumed an average of 2,450 calories a day. In the 2005-08 survey, men consumed an average of 2,656 calories a day. Women increased their caloric intake by almost 300 calories during the same time period. In the 1971-74 survey, women consumed approximately 1,542 calories a day. In the 2005-08 survey, women consumed an average of 1,811 calories a day. During that time the percentage of calories from protein, total fat, and saturated fat has decreased, while the percentage of calories from carbohydrates has increased. [14]

This can be partially explained by the price of food as a percentage of our income. Because of increased efficiency in food production and distribution and increased spending power, we spend less on food as a percentage of our income. We spent 23.2 percent of our income on food in 1968.[15] In 2008, food as a percentage of income was 11.4 percent.[16] Food is cheap and plentiful. Even better, quick, fattening foods are at every corner, and they crowd our grocery store shelves.

Additionally, we are more sedentary than we were forty years ago. In the past, we worked manual labor jobs that required more physical energy and longer hours. The percentage of persons working in farming, manufacturing, construction, and mining has decreased from 36.7 percent in 1970[17] to 21 percent in 2009.[18] We require fewer calories to do our job, and we have more time to eat. We live farther away from grocery stores and shopping centers, so we drive more and walk less. We use escalators instead of stairs. Airports have shuttles and moving walkways. Cell phones and computers have changed how we communicate. What's the point in walking to a neighbor's house or meeting at a park when you can simply send a text message?

The cost of our overindulgence is staggering. The Center for Disease Control and Prevention estimated the health care costs for overweight and obese people to be more than $147 billion in 2008. Since then, we have not become thinner, and the cost of health care has not decreased.

Steve and Beth weren't concerned about health care costs or surveys at the moment. They arrived at the hotel and checked in. The resort hotel was an older place, but with its lazy river pool, view of the mountains, and central location, it had managed to remain a popular destination. Located in the north part of Phoenix, it was only a few miles from Steve's old high school.

Even though their room wasn't far from the front desk, they accepted a ride to it in a golf cart. They rode past the regular rooms and turned left just beyond a cowboy-themed restaurant. They saw Steve's classmate Matt walking in the same direction, pulling his wheeled suitcase.

"Hey, Matt, what's going on?" Steve said. Steve and Matt hadn't been good friends in high school, but they had hung out at the twenty-year reunion and had become Facebook® friends. Matt's hairline had receded since the last reunion, but he also looked as if he had lost some weight.

"Hi, Steve," Matt replied. "Glad to see you made it. I was hoping it wasn't just the pinheads who came." He couldn't remember Beth's name, and neither Steve nor Beth offered it.

"What are you doing walking?" Steve said. "Hop in. We'll give you a ride."

Matt smiled. "Thanks, but I'm okay walking." "It's not too far from here. You guys heading to the restaurant tonight for the festivities?"

"Yep," Steve said. "See you there."

They had rented a bi-level casita with a living room and kitchenette on the bottom floor and a master bedroom on the second floor. It was decorated in a southwestern style, complete with an old fireplace and southwest landscape paintings in all the rooms. They had a private patio in the back with a view of the mountain preserve.

Steve stretched out on the couch and turned on the television. Beth explored the rooms. They had a couple of hours before they headed to the restaurant. In the past there was no doubt what they would be doing. But Steve was tired. Lately it seemed as if Steve was always tired. Within fifteen minutes he was snoring.

Beth had seen it coming. In the past, she would have been angry about wasting an opportunity without the kids around. But her moods had shifted from tired to irritable. She just shrugged and called home to let them know that they had arrived safely and to see how they were doing.

Sara was easy to deal with. She was still young and liked spending time with her parents. She was a few years from puberty, or so Beth hoped, and her innocence was refreshing.

Zack was a petulant fifteen-year-old who couldn't understand the need for a baby-sitter. They had switched schools last year so that Zack could play baseball on a team that was known to produce professional players. Unfortunately, the coach had it in for Zack, and he didn't make the team. At least that was Steve's theory. Zack was despondent. He still had club baseball, but not playing for his high school baseball team was difficult.

Ronda had recently graduated from the University of Washington and was working downtown as a paralegal until she figured out her next move. As a parent you think eighteen is some magic number. Technically, you are no longer responsible for your children once they reach that age. As Beth hung up the phone she thought that being a worried parent had no age limit.

Steve and Beth used the golf cart to go to the restaurant for the Friday night gathering. It was a casual affair, so Steve wore jeans and a light blue button-down shirt. Beth wore a pair of khaki Capri pants and a red floral top. It was cold for Phoenicians but closer to summer weather for Beth.

About halfway there, they saw Matt walking on the sidewalk toward the restaurant.

"What is this? Are you swearing off mechanized transportation?" Steve said. "Get your butt in the cart!"

Matt hesitated but decided it would be rude to refuse. "Sure, why not," Matt replied as he climbed into the cart.

"Seriously, Matt, we're about three quarters of a mile from the restaurant. Why didn't you call for transportation?"

"I don't know if you noticed, but I lost about thirty pounds since our last reunion."

"I thought you looked thinner," Beth said. Steve eyed Beth but didn't say anything.

"Have you ever heard of Non-Exercise Activity Thermogenesis, or NEAT?" asked Matt.

Steve and Beth shook their head.

"NEAT is defined as the energy expenditure of all physical activities other than exercise done on purpose.[19]    Such activities include 'fidgeting, spontaneous muscle contraction, and maintaining posture when not recumbent.' [20]  In other words, anything done when not lying down or not purposefully exercising is defined as NEAT.

"I consider NEAT an easy calorie burner." Matt continued. "The more I looked into NEAT, the clearer it became that we have an infinite number of ways to burn extra calories without jumping onto a treadmill.  In fact, studies show that NEAT is capable of limiting fat gain even in situations where people are overfed by as much as a thousand calories a day.[21]

Steve thought about the dreaded treadmill and smiled.

"The number of calories expended in non-exercise activity varies dramatically depending on occupational duties and leisure activity.  Your occupation can have a great influence on how many calories you expend.  A construction worker or anyone who works in a job that requires physical activity can expend 50 percent more calories than an office worker." [22]

"Maybe that's why I began to gain weight after I got my desk job," Steve said.

"It could be, but you probably aren't going to beg your boss for a demotion," Matt said.  "Besides, your leisure activity can also impact your caloric expenditure.  The couch potato may use a thousand fewer calories than the person who chooses to walk to work, walk the dog, or perform some other physical activities.[23]

"Researchers tested ten lean, sedentary volunteers and ten sedentary, slightly obese volunteers for the amount of time they spent lying down, sitting, and standing.  The lean volunteers spent approximately two and a half hours more time on their feet than the obese volunteers.  The researchers noted that had the obese volunteers spent as much time on their feet as the lean volunteers, they would have expended an additional three hundred and fifty calories a day.[24] Over a year, this would have resulted in a loss of more than twenty pounds had they eaten the same amount."

"Wow!" Beth exclaimed.

"There is evidence that the relationship between obesity and the expenditure of calories in everyday life is profound," Matt continued. "The studies limited the amount of exercise in order to reveal the effects of NEAT on weight gain and obesity. In all of the studies, the researchers found a direct relationship between NEAT and obesity. The more calories used in NEAT, the less likely someone was going to be obese."

"That sounds like a bunch of crap to me," Steve said, looking skeptical.

"I agree, it sounds a little screwy," Matt said. "But it worked for me. I wasn't a couch potato before, but I would find the closest parking space even if I had to wait, and I would take the elevator instead of the stairs. Frankly, I found NEAT to be a simple concept where small changes made a big difference. I didn't change my life dramatically, but I made a few changes that have become part of my daily routine and helped me lose the thirty pounds and keep it off."

"Like walking instead of taking the golf cart," Steve said.

"Yes, like walking instead of taking the golf cart. I also park farther away from stores, I garden instead of watching television, I stand up when I would normally be seated, I pace when I'm on the phone, I wash my own car, and I take stairs instead of the elevator," Matt said "I lost thirty pounds over a two-year period, and I have managed to keep it off for the last three years."

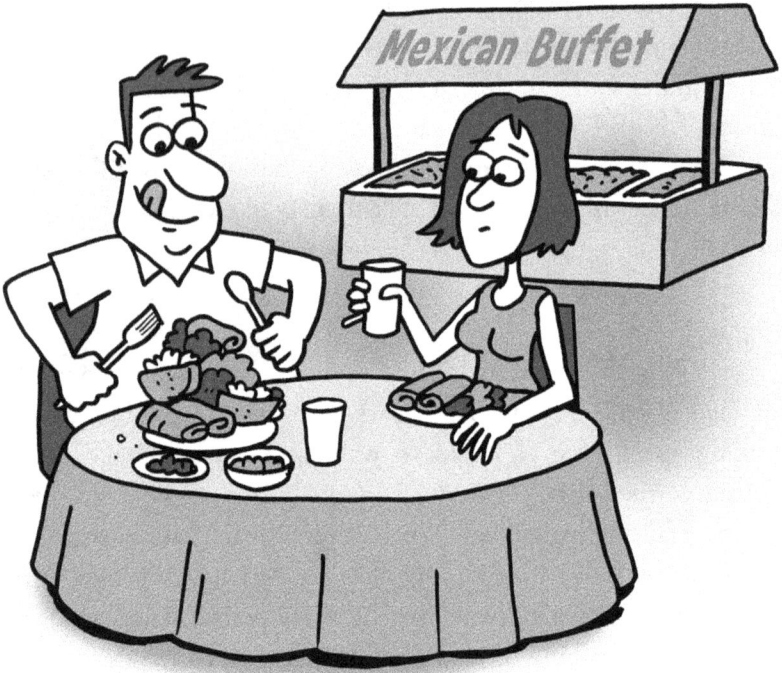

# 4

## HOW DID I GET THIS FULL?

They arrived at the restaurant. It was a Mexican restaurant built like an adobe house, with a front patio and a cabana-style bar, plus a saloon-style bar inside, where they had live music, and a large outdoor bar and back patio. The reunion committee had set up a buffet there.

Beth, Steve, and Matt grabbed drinks and headed toward the gathering. Beth hesitated. She knew that she was an hour away from being alone in the crowd. Every reunion, every gathering, was the same. Steve and his buddies got a few drinks in them and recalled their misspent youth. She had heard the same stories for years. The only things that changed were the narrators' girth and hairline and the looks of the women they had romanced and the size of the foes they had conquered. Eventually, she would be left to her own resources. Fortunately, she wasn't shy, and she was always able to entertain herself. But it was still annoying.

Steve headed straight to the buffet. He hadn't eaten since they left Seattle, and he was starving. He loaded his plate with three beef enchiladas, rice, refried beans, and sour cream. He added a couple of sopapillas so he could get his sugar fix. Then he found a table with a couple of his classmates and their spouses already dining.

He sat between Ivan and Marcia. She was a fellow classmate of Steve's. Seven years ago she and her husband had undergone gastric bypass surgery. They were both morbidly obese and felt that surgery was their best bet for getting control of their weight.

Surgery is often a means of last resort when diet programs fail. It seemed as if there are as many diets as there are foods. Do a quick search on the Internet, and you will find hundreds if not thousands of sites claiming they have the answer to your weight problem. Some diets require you to eat certain types of foods, while others ask you to avoid certain foods. Medifast®, Jenny Craig®, and other similar diets offer their food as a way of limiting your caloric intake. Other diets insist that you avoid sugar or processed foods or meat.

A relatively new diet called the caveman diet has its advocates. The idea behind this diet is that you eat only what you could get by hunting, fishing, and foraging the way prehistoric people did before we domesticated animals and developed agriculture. It seems odd to advocate eating the way people who lived short, brutal lives did, when food intake ranged from gorging after a kill to near starvation when food was scarce. But if it works, great!

There are also a number of hypo-caloric diets where the calorie intake is well below the daily caloric needs. These are diets that should be performed only under the supervision of a doctor. The HCG diet, for example, requires you to limit your caloric intake to as few as 500 calories (called a hypo-caloric diet) while injecting HCG, a hormone produced during pregnancy. The HCG hormone is supposed to suppress hunger and increase fat loss over muscle loss during the program. People have lost thirty or forty pounds during one course of an HCG diet. Another hypo-caloric diet limits your carbohydrate intake to the point where your body must use fat as its source of energy (called ketosis). Again, this is a medically supervised diet that has shown weight loss of as much as a pound a day.

In some instances, surgical procedures may be the answer for morbidly obese people. Morbidly obese is defined as either a BMI of over forty for a male who is more than 100 pounds overweight or a female who is more than eighty pounds overweight.[25]

Before consenting to surgery, Ivan and Marcia were required to participate in a psychological evaluation to determine their ability to adhere to a very strict eating regimen after the procedure. Because your stomach is smaller after the surgery, you can eat only small portions. In essence, it forces you to change your eating habits. But even surgery offers no guarantee of long-term success.

Steve had last seen Ivan and Marcia at the twenty-year reunion, two years after they had surgery. They were much thinner then, and they appeared to be on their way to a healthy life. Unfortunately, Ivan was back to his old weight or maybe even heavier. Steve was stunned.

"Hi, Steve, hi, Beth," Marcia said. "How are you?"

Marcia had sat down just before Steve did, but it looked as if she had eaten on her way to the table, because her food covered a little more than half the plate. She had turned the whole beans, rice, lettuce, tomatoes, salsa, and chicken into a salad. Ivan was not as creative. He had heaped his plate with food, even more than Steve had.

"We're doing well," Steve replied. "We're happy to get out of the rain for a few days. How are you guys doing?"

"Not too great, Steve," Ivan said before Marcia could respond. "That surgery didn't do a thing for me." It took Ivan a few seconds to complete the last sentence because he was busy shoveling food into his mouth, as if there was a looming famine that only he knew about.

Ivan was a stark reminder that even surgery is no guarantee of success without a change in behavior. In a study comparing extremely obese individuals who went on a conventional diet versus a surgical procedure, those who underwent surgery ate more fat, fast food, and less breakfast than the nonsurgical participants. Nonsurgical participants spent more time in physical activity. Both surgical and nonsurgical participants who were successful at maintaining their weight loss reported high levels of physical activity. Surgical participants reported higher levels of depression and stress than nonsurgical participants. It appears that for all participants, the susceptibility to losing control over their eating habits played the greatest role in weight regain.[26]

"It worked for me," Marcia said, ignoring Ivan. "They shrink the stomach from about a quart to two ounces. They place you on a liquid diet that evolves into a low-fat, high-protein diet. You have to avoid sugary foods because of their high-calorie content and because they pass too quickly through your stomach, a process called 'dumping,' which can cause cramping, nausea, and diarrhea. We had to take vitamin and mineral supplements and to stay hydrated, and we had to eat smaller meals. And, because our stomachs were so small, we were forced to limit our intake.

"It was difficult at first, but I got used to the small portions," Marcia said. "You have to drink water between meals and chew your food slowly. Those three instructions——eat smaller portions (no meal bigger than your fist), drink water, and chew slowly——have helped me control my weight. The gastric bypass surgery was the force that helped me lose weight, but I'm convinced that my lifestyle change is what's keeping it off."

Steve looked at Ivan. Obviously, the lifestyle change did not work for him.

"Ivan is a seafood eater," Marcia said. "When he sees food, he eats it. We didn't understand at the time of the surgery that your stomach can expand. I think Ivan looked at it as a miracle cure. Initially it was. But Ivan's portions grew and grew to the point that I think he ate as much as he did before. As it turned out, the ability to resist opportunities to overeat and control or regulate your dietary intake are strong predictors of weight-loss maintenance." [27]

"I want to kick the crap out of those doctors," Ivan said, clenching his fists. "For a while I could eat in small portions and feel full. Now I feel hungry all the time. I realize it worked great for Marcia, and I'm happy for her. But it was no miracle cure for me. To tell you the truth, it's just very disheartening."

Steve didn't say anything. He had almost lost his appetite. But his love for Mexican food and his vast hunger overcame his impulse to stop eating. He wolfed down his food and excused himself, claiming he needed another drink.

Steve had already abandoned Beth. She wasn't surprised and was in fact enjoying herself. She sat next to Ken and Laurie. Laurie was Steve's classmate. She was also a dentist who recently moved back from Albuquerque. Ken was a recent boyfriend. Laurie had a sharp tongue and the ability to comment on the decline of her classmates, including herself, in a way that was very funny without offending anyone.

While Steve stood at the bar, Doug came up to him and said, "Hey, Steve, how's life in the rain forest?" Doug was a Phoenix police officer. If what they say about cops and donuts is true, Doug did not get the memo. He was Doug's height but looked the way Steve had when Steve was twenty-five.

He and Steve had known each other ever since they played Pop Warner football in the fifth grade. They also played football together in high school and kept in touch. He considered asking Doug how he stayed in shape but decided that Doug would just laugh at him and give him a bunch of crap.

"Beats the desert," Steve said. "Where's Nancy?"

"Nancy hates these events," Doug replied, referring to his wife. "She says it's a bunch of fat old people lying about their past to people they once knew. I told her not to leave me alone with all these hot women who I had a crush on." They both laughed.

Steve and Doug began the ritualistic reminiscing. Steve tried to concentrate on the conversation, but the plate and a half of food had made him feel stuffed and groggy. His body was trying to digest the cheese, tortilla, refried beans, rice, sautéed beef, sour cream, and beer he had just consumed.

"Sorry, Doug, I have to sit down," Steve said. "I'm feeling stuffed and tired from all the Mexican food I ate."

Doug laughed. "I'm not surprised. You just ate enough to feed a family of four for a day."

"What are you talking about? I haven't eaten all day, and I was starving. My body obviously needed the food or I wouldn't have been so hungry."

"You may know how to wire a house, but you obviously don't know anything about how our bodies work."

"What's to know? You get hungry, and you eat. It seems pretty simple to me."

Doug laughed again. "Well, as your gut tries to get its arms around your simple food, let me explain how our digestive system really works."

"As we sit here fat and happy, inside our bodies are large industrial complexes where cells are destroyed and rebuilt. With hundreds of millions of workers, the breakdown and buildup, often referred to as metabolism, is an extremely complex process, with billions of cells in constant motion. The brain manages the process by sending chemical instructions to various systems, organs, hormones, and glands. The process requires energy not unlike a car needs gasoline and air to run. However, the body is far more complicated than an internal combustion engine and, as such, it requires a wide variety of energy sources that we supply when we eat, drink, and breathe.

"While we can survive for quite some time without food— prisoners have lived more than ten weeks with only water— ultimately, we need food to supply our body with the energy it needs. How much food we need depends on our energy level, our size, the climate where we exist, and our body's need to rebuild itself. In a perfect system, our brain through our various organs and hormones relays the amount and variety of food we eat. We, in turn, go to the grocery store or restaurant and order the foods our body requires and eat the amount and variety it needs."

Steve chuckled, thinking about the variety of food he ate when he was hungry. He wanted to ask how many food groups are in a pepperoni pizza but didn't.

"Sounds great, and to some degree that's how it works," Doug continued. "When we're hungry our body secretes hormones that tell our brain that we need food. When we're full our body produces hormones that let our body know that it has had enough to eat. In theory, the system works great. But what happens when you're hungry and you don't take the time to eat? Or, like most people, you eat only two or three times a day regardless of what your body is telling you.

"I ate a little something for breakfast this morning," Steve admitted. "But that was it."

"Exactly! You didn't eat until well after your body asked for food. By the time you got to the buffet, it had been a few hours since you last ate. It was panic time for your body. It acted as if it may never see food again. It craved the foods that would last through the next famine. Those are foods high in fat for storage and foods high in sugars for instant energy.

"You inhaled a meal with well over a thousand calories, more than half your daily caloric needs, in minutes. Marcia had less than a third of the calories, with a lot more nutritional value."

"How did I have three times more calories than Marcia?"

"First, you ate more than she did. She didn't feel the need to fill her plate. She had less than half the amount of food that you had. You both had grilled chicken, rice, lettuce, and tomatoes. Depending on how the rice was processed, that's a pretty decent meal."

"And beans," Steve said.

"You both had beans, but she had whole beans, and you had refried beans. Whole beans are high in fiber and protein without adding a lot of calories. Refried beans add oil or lard and can double the number of calories.

"She added salsa, which is a mix of tomatoes, spices, and water. Her salsa added flavoring but not many calories. You added tortillas, cheese, and sour cream. The tortilla was reprocessed flour or a simple carbohydrate devoid of nutritional value but high in calories. Cheese is a high-calorie concentration of fat and protein, and sour cream is pure fat. Finally, you ate a sopapilla with honey, adding even more calories with a large amount of sugar."

Steve was amazed. No wonder he was stuffed. He had never put any thought into his food. He just ate it. Marcia weighed almost 100 pounds more than he did seven years ago. Now she weighed 100 pounds less. Could the difference in weight change be due to her eating habits versus his?

"Where was I?" Doug said. "Oh, yeah. Your digestive system goes to work trying to process the food. Energy resources are sent to the stomach and intestine. The various hormones in charge of managing food digestion work in overdrive. You far exceeded your body's current needs, but the body has a motto. 'Waste not, want not.' Nutrients not activated for immediate needs are placed in storage for the next famine. This is easy, since you ate foods abundant in fat and simple carbohydrates that the body finds easy to store."

Steve looked down at his engorged stomach. It was not uncommon for him to skip a meal and then drive to the nearest fast food restaurant and order the greasiest food on the menu.

"Of course most of us don't need to be hungry to eat," Doug added. "Most family celebrations revolve around food. Your daughter wins her basketball game, so how about some ice cream now? You get back to work, and it's time to celebrate Martha's birthday with a cake. We eat when we're happy, and we eat when we're sad or depressed. Unfortunately, we never eat vegetables, fruits, nuts, or fish in those situations. We gravitate toward foods high in fat or sugar."

"Heck, I'll eat a bag of chips as I watch television," Steve confessed. "I've been eating like crap for years."

Doug laughed. "Well, you know how it works, Steve. Positive change comes with knowing what you need to do to make the change and then doing it."

Doug decided to change the subject by pointing to Angie, one of their former classmates. "Angie looks as good now as she did when she was eighteen," Doug said.

Steve looked at her. "I had illegal thoughts about her when we were in high school. Even if I wasn't married, I can't say I'd be able to do much with her now."

"Why don't you get your testosterone levels checked? Testosterone is associated with libido, mood, lean muscle tissue, and bone mineral density in men and women. Those levels decline as we age.[28] I have a bunch of friends who get shots for it."

"I don't know, Doug. It seems pretty intrusive just for an increased sex drive."

"Testosterone isn't just about that. First, there is some evidence that erectile dysfunction may be a predictor of Metabolic Syndrome. An analysis of studies on testosterone and Metabolic Syndrome showed that patients with Metabolic Syndrome have lower plasma levels of testosterone. Those levels appear to be specifically linked to insulin resistance. Subjects who received testosterone replacement reduced some of their symptoms of Metabolic Syndrome.[29] So just for that reason, you should look into it.

"Second, low testosterone may lead to depression and decreased cognitive function. I would personally attest to your doctor that you are showing signs of both based on your disinterest in sex."

Steve laughed aloud, but he thought about his recent issues with Beth.

"How do I get this tested?"

"Go to a doctor. He'll run a battery of tests. I went to check it out because some of my buddies told me their workouts were better. But the doctor told me I was fine."

"I'll look into it," Steve said. "Maybe I'll be able to bench press my weight."

Doug smiled. "That would be impressive."

Doug excused himself as Beth approached the bar.

"Was that Doug?" Beth asked.

"Yes. He was telling me how our digestive system works and how I shouldn't wait to eat because that makes me hungry for lots of heavy foods."

"I saw that Marcia ate smaller portions and left out the tortillas and the sour cream," Beth said. "Maybe we should try and limit our meal size and eat more often."

"I also I like Matt's suggestion to stand more, do more physically active hobbies, and walk instead of drive whenever it's feasible," Steve said.

"Yes, I really think the NEAT concept is great," Beth agreed.

"Between Doug and Matt's advice, it was an informative evening," Steve said.

The remaining evening went as Beth had expected. Most of the locals drifted away. Beth left around 10:30. She was tired, and she was hearing too much about how cool and virile the men were "back in the day." Steve remained there until closing time.

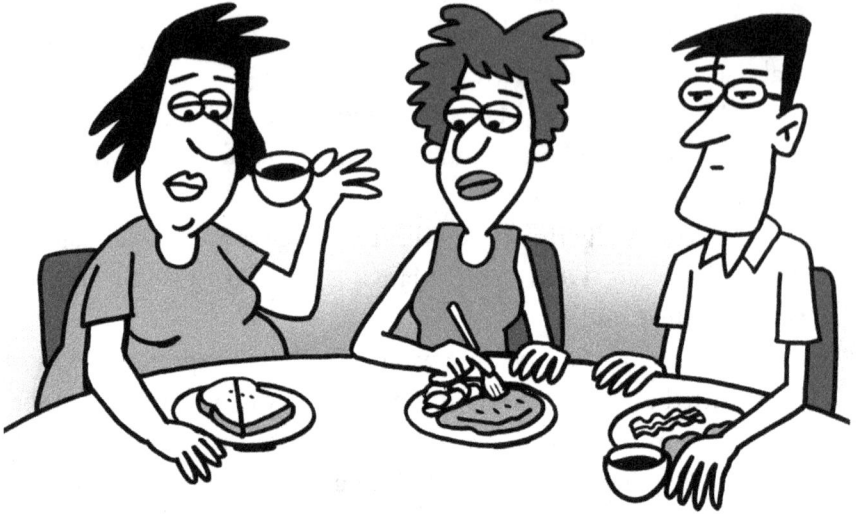

# 5

## GLUTEN AND FOOD ALLERGIES

Beth went to breakfast alone. She was an early riser and knew that after a late night out, Steve would want to sleep in. She decided to take Matt's advice and walk down to the lobby restaurant instead of taking a cart. The host was about to seat her when she heard someone call her name. It was Laurie, the dentist, and Ken.

"Come sit with us, Beth," Laurie said. "Where's your lout of a husband? Last time I saw him he and Matt were having a foot race from the restaurant to the casitas. After about seventy-five yards Matt was going backward and Steve was doubled over, cursing him. Steve was forced to walk the rest of the way with his pants down around his ankles. I never pictured him as a boxers guy."

Beth chuckled. Normally she would have found this hilarious, but with the news from the doctor it didn't seem as amusing.

The waiter came to take their order. Ken chose the buffet, and Laurie ordered a vegetable omelet without cheese and the fruit plate. Beth ordered a coffee and sour dough toast.

"That's a tough way to start your morning," Laurie said to Beth.

"What do you mean? I always drink coffee in the morning," Beth replied, feeling slightly offended.

"I wasn't talking about your coffee. I was talking about how little you're eating and how devoid of nutrients your breakfast is."

"I'm just not hungry in the morning," Beth said. "Besides, what's wrong with toast?"

"First, sour dough bread is only slightly better for you than eating straight sugar. The coffee and the toast will give you a boost of energy for about an hour, and then you'll get tired and very hungry. I have found that having some protein such as an egg white and foods with fiber like whole fruit help my energy level and keep me from feeling famished by eleven."

"Second, I've been gluten-free for about two years," Laurie added.

"Gluten-free? I've heard of that but don't know what it is. It seems like one of those fad diets."

"I don't think it's a diet, and I don't know if it's a fad. I just know that it works for me," Laurie said. "I felt tired and run down all the time, so I saw a doctor, but he couldn't find anything wrong with me. I began researching my issues online. A lot of research is done on menopause and our bodies' response to it. Since I'm not at that stage of my life, I knew it had to be something else. My ex-husband just thought it was a 'female problem.'"

Laurie looked right at Ken. "They call them ex-husbands for a reason."

"Anyway, a friend of mine told me to research food allergies. She thought maybe my sense of malaise was caused by something I was eating. So I researched food allergies.[30]

"The most common food allergies accounting for about 90 percent of the reactions are milk, eggs, peanuts, soy, shellfish, fish, wheat, and tree nuts. [31] Food allergies provoke an immune system response where you may have a runny nose or watery eyes. Under certain circumstances you may have difficulty breathing." [32]

"A friend of mine has something like that," Beth said. "She carries an inhaler, and if a food has an ingredient in it that she's allergic to and she moves around too much after eating it, she has trouble breathing."

"She has food-dependent, exercise-induced anaphylaxis," Laurie said. Whatever that means, Beth thought.

"Yes, I know that's quite a mouthful, Laurie said. Food intolerance refers to a non-allergic reaction to food, either due to something in the food or something in the person that responds to the food. Symptoms include fatigue, headache, and irritable bowel. The reaction doesn't always manifest itself immediately, so it's difficult to diagnose. It can result from the body not producing an enzyme that responds to a particular food item, a toxic reaction, or chronic infections.

"A common reason for food intolerance is carbohydrate malabsorption such as lactose intolerance, where lactose cannot be absorbed in the small intestine because of a deficiency in the enzyme lactase. Similar problems may occur with the inability to absorb other carbohydrates such as fructose or sorbitol, a sugar alcohol found in many fruits."[33],[34]

"But how about wheat? Beth asked. "We've been eating wheat for as long as we've been growing our own food. Now some quack decides that all our problems stem from my beloved bread?

"You're right, we've been eating wheat for over ten thousand years. It's currently grown in over a hundred countries, and it's a primary source of protein, iron, zinc, and selenium.[35] However, wheat is also one of the eight foods associated with food allergies, and it's part of a recent phenomenon known as gluten intolerance. Gluten, a protein, gives wheat a binding affect that makes it good for making dough for breads and pastas.[36] Extreme gluten intolerance is called celiac disease.[37]

"However, gluten sensitivity is defined as the body's inability to properly break down and absorb a protein found in gluten. This causes an inflammatory reaction that may eventually cause celiac disease.

Even if it doesn't, ongoing gluten sensitivity can cause organ damage, tissue damage, and auto-immune disease.[38]

"The fact is there are no definitive tests that tell us if we're gluten-intolerant," Laurie continued. "Most of the evidence regarding gluten intolerance is anecdotal. If you  went to a doctor with symptoms ranging from  feeling run down or depressed, or having a low sex drive, they would do some blood tests, but at your age we can assume you are menopausal or perimenopausal. They may check your thyroid and your hormones and prescribe a thyroid medication or hormone therapy. Or they may just tell you to get used to it.

"You may not have a food allergy or intolerance, but if you're feeling crappy, looking at your food as a possible culprit is easier and less invasive than stuffing pills down your throat.  And it beats resigning yourself to living in a funk."

Beth looked at the remaining piece of toast on her plate. She loved bread and couldn't imagine giving it up.  But she hated feeling like this.  She decided to do her own research and ask around when she got back to Seattle.

They spent another half hour watching people picking up food items, looking at them, and replacing them. Laurie found the spectacle to be amusing.  But Beth and Ken thought the food handling was disgusting.

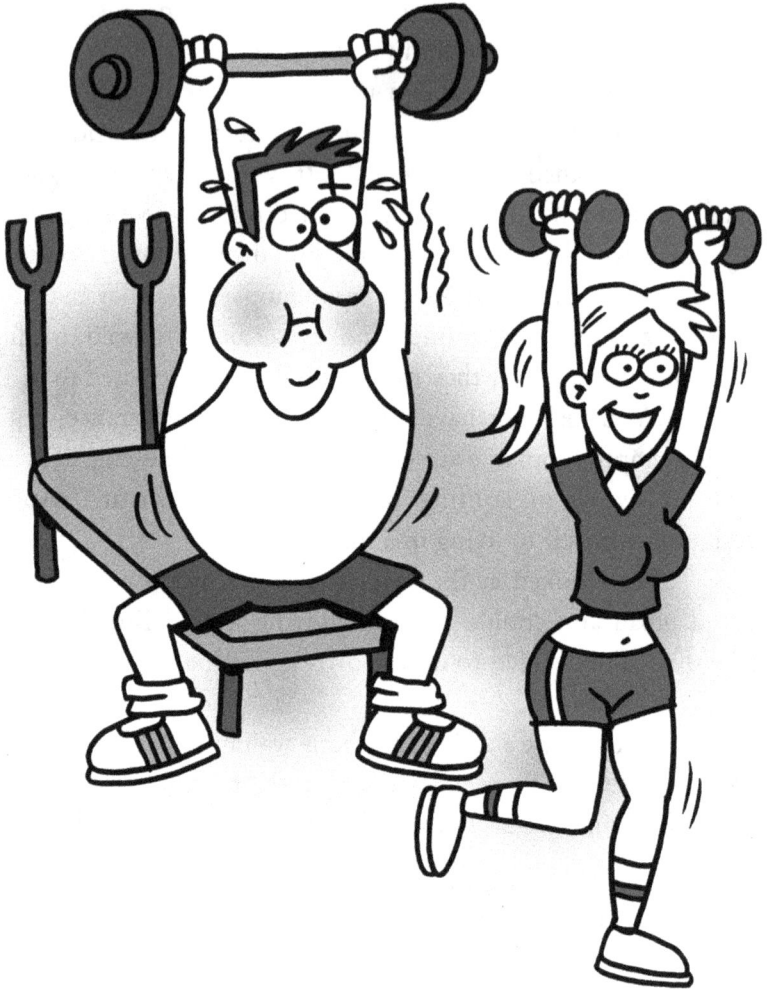

# 6

## RESISTANCE TRAINING

Steve rolled out of bed around nine. Cobwebs filled his head. He grabbed a soda out of the mini-fridge and tried to recall the prior evening. The rewind stopped at his race with Matt. He was laughing at the time, but now he felt embarrassed. How did I get this out of shape? he thought. He didn't have an answer. He snatched a candy bar from the fridge, threw on some clothes, and headed out the door.

He was wandering toward the main lobby when he spied the gym. On a whim he decided to check it out. It was similar to many resort gyms. Treadmills, elliptical machines, and stationary bikes faced a large mirror, with televisions in front of and above each machine. Two benches and a few free weights sat in the corner. The rest of the first room consisted of rows of Nautilus machines. The back room had padded floors, a mirror that lined one end, and a mat and small dumbbells along the side.

It had been a long time since he worked out. He wasn't even sure what he would do in a gym. He was about to leave when he heard someone say his name.

"Hey, Steve, you looking to challenge someone else to a foot race?" It was Rob, another classmate. He had run track and cross country in high school. Steve expected to see him on the treadmill, but to Steve's surprise Rob sat at an upright bench press.

"Hey, Rob!" Steve replied. "No thanks. One butt kicking a weekend is my limit. But I am looking for the jerk who over-served me last night. What are you doing at a weight machine? I figured to see you on a treadmill."

"Do you think I'm getting too bulky?" Rob laughed, flexing his slender but well defined arm. "I try to do some form of resistance training at least twice a week to maintain or at least limit muscle loss as I get older."

"What's resistance training? Do you mean weight lifting?"

"Weight lifting is one form of resistance training or strength training," Rob said. "Other forms of resistance training include using your own body as resistance such as doing push-ups or pull-ups, free weights, weight training machines such as Nautilus equipment, resistance bands, or any other means of physical pressure applied against an external force."

"I can't see the point of resistance training," Steve said. "I need to lose weight, not bulk up."

"Resistance training uses calories, so it'll help you lose weight. But it's just one of many factors when it comes to weight loss and weight maintenance."

"Matt was telling me about how he increased his caloric use just by doing more walking and standing and doing more physically demanding hobbies. I think he called it NEAT."

"I know a little bit about NEAT. I think it has some validity, but I also know if you want to lose weight, or even not gain weight, you need to exercise more and eat less."

"I know that people who run tend to by thinner," Steve said, "but I really don't know why."

Rob finished his bench presses and sat down to perform another exercise. "Do you know what metabolism is?"

"The doctor mentioned it, but I don't think I know what it means."

"You don't see it when looking in the mirror," Rob said, "but your body is in a constant state of breaking down and rebuilding itself. The process is called metabolism. This process requires energy. Calories are a measure of the energy we take in, as food and drink, and the energy we use as we move around, digest our food, and as our bodies rebuild themselves. As I said, weight control has two sides—the intake side or what you eat and drink as measured in calories, and the outtake side or how your body uses those calories.

"Most people think of burning calories in terms of exercise, but your body is constantly burning them. Your daily caloric use can be broken down into three areas: the calories you need to subsist, called Basal Metabolic Rate or Resting Metabolic Rate, the calories you need to digest your food, called diet-induced thermogenesis, and the calories you need to move, called activity thermogenesis.

"First, I have some positive news."

Steve stared at Rob. He could use some positive news.

"Even at complete rest your body continues to work," Rob explained. "Your heart is beating, you're breathing, and your brain continues to function. Besides that, your muscles, skin, kidneys, liver, and other internal organs are breaking down and rebuilding cells. This requires energy. In fact, about 60 percent of your daily calories are used in this process. This number is mostly related to your lean body mass, or your fat-free body weight. The number of calories used in this process is called the basal metabolic rate, or BMR.

"So guess what? You can lose weight while sleeping or watching television! The next time you get hooked on an exercise infomercial, pay attention to whether they mention the calories you burn after exercising or while you sleep after using their contraption for less than half an hour a week. When they mention calories burned after exercise, they're referring to either the energy used to recover from the exercise or the energy increase due to the increased muscle mass you accumulated during your workout.

"BMR is the energy you use when at rest. It may seem counterintuitive to think that you have some control over your internal workings as you rest or sleep. But you do. BMR is related to your fat-free muscle mass. The most effective way to increase your basal metabolic rate is to increase your fat-free mass. You do that by increasing your muscle mass."

"Is that why you're working out?"

"It is one of the reasons."

"How do I know what my BMR is?"

"If you ever want a true measure of the calories you're burning at rest, it's measured twelve hours after you last ate so that it doesn't measure the calories needed to digest a meal. Of course the measurement requires expensive equipment that you probably don't have. But you can find a way to estimate your BMR online. It will ask for your weight, height, age, and sex. Since lean body mass is a strong predictor of BMR, online BMR estimates predict your fat-free body weight and calculate the number of calories required, based on that prediction.

"Women tend to have more fat than men, so BMR is lower for women of the same weight and height. We normally lose muscle as we age, so any predictive model will lower BMR because of that. Finally, your height and weight are used to estimate your lean body mass. At five-four and a hundred and forty pounds, a forty-five-year-old female will have an estimated BMR of a little over thirteen hundred calories. A five-ten, hundred and eighty- pound, forty-four- year-old male will have an estimated BMR of a little over seventeen hundred calories."

"I remember a hundred and eighty pounds about a thousand cheeseburgers ago," Steve said, rubbing his stomach.

Rob laughed. "Which thousand do you think did it?"

Steve didn't find the question as humorous as Rob did.

"Your BMR decreases as you age," Rob continued. "While you may link this to your diminished energy levels or your body slowing down, it is most likely a result of a decrease in muscle mass. On average we lose eighteen percent of our muscle mass between the age of twenty and fifty and an additional twenty percent between the age of fifty and eighty." [39]

"How do you increase your muscle mass?" Rob asked.

"Resistance training?"

"Exactly!"

"The second way you use calories is to digest your food," Rob said.

"Heck, Rob if food digestion is a weight-loss regimen, count me in."

"But unless you eat only cabbage or celery, you're out of luck."

"Your digestive system starts processing the food and liquid you ingest from the moment it enters your mouth. Some of your hormones, such as insulin, increase at the mere thought of food. Digestion requires calories to break down your food into smaller particles, which are either used in your body for cell regeneration or other needs, or they're sent through our digestive system and end up as waste. Food digestion requires approximately a hundred and fifty to two hundred and fifty calories a day or six to twelve percent of the calories used in a day."

All this talk about food is making Steve hungry. He and Matt are meeting at a local diner for lunch. He thought about what Doug said about the body and how it reacts when it's in starvation mode, but he decided to ignore his hunger pangs and wait to eat until lunchtime.

"So I'm using calories at rest and after eating," Steve said.

"That's right. But wait, there's more!" They both laughed.

"The remaining daily calorie use is through activity thermogenesis or any activity other than rest or digestion," Rob explained. "Activity thermogenesis is broken down into two additional categories: the first one is NEAT, the one Matt told you about. I won't dispute that NEAT is a great way to burn calories, but for a variety of reasons I think the second category, exercise, is more important."

"Exercise includes activities such as running, biking, lifting weights, and taking part in sports or any other physical activity done at least in part to become or remain physically fit. While I'm a big fan of aerobic exercise, resistance training has a number of fantastic benefits. It reduces muscle mass loss as you age, increases your basal metabolic rate, increases the number of calories you use during and after the training session, positively affects certain hormones, and improves functional capacity."

Steve's phone rang.

"Hold that thought," Steve told Rob.

"Hey, Beth, what's up?"

Beth said that she had called Ronda to check in. Everything was fine on the home front. Ronda had ordered pizza last night. Sara spent the night on her computer, and Zack spent it in his room watching television. Steve thought about Sara. She had gained weight lately. He worried about making her too aware of it because he was afraid she'd develop an eating disorder. But she was spending more time on her computer and less time playing outside. He made a mental note to see how his eating and exercise habits might be affecting his kids.

Steve pocketed his phone and apologized for the interruption.

"No big deal," Rob replied. "I always say 'you have two responsibilities in life—one to yourself and one to your family. Mess up one and the other one won't matter.'"

Steve nodded in agreement and looked into a mirror. He wondered if he was bequeathing an unhealthy, sedentary lifestyle to his kids. He shook the thought off, looked at Rob, and said "Where were we?"

"We were talking about avoiding sarcopenia," Rob replied.

"I thought we were talking about resistance training."

"We were. Sarcopenia is the name given to the progressive loss of muscle mass and strength as we age.[40] The first muscles to go are the type two muscles, or fast-twitch muscles. Even if you aren't a sprinter, everyone has fast-twitch muscles. These are the primary muscles used in lifting or quick movements. As we age, these muscles are converted to slow-twitch muscles. This decreases our functional capacity--our ability to complete basic daily activities.

"Some muscle loss is inevitable. We can't be twenty again. We will always search for the fountain of youth, but as of now, we are bound by the forces of nature."

"No kidding," Steve said, looking at a young man working out with free weights. He was a reflection of himself twenty years earlier. He looked into a mirror and sucked in his gut.

"While some muscle loss is not irreversible, exercise can slow the atrophy," Rob said. "Resistance training has been shown to increase muscle mass by over eleven percent and muscle strength by over a hundred percent. Positive results have been shown in as little as two days a week of thirty- minute sessions."[41],[42]

Steve thought about his pathetic foot race the night before. In high school and college he had been a fast runner. He pictured his type two muscles abandoning him as he abandoned exercise.

"Another benefit to resistance training is that increases in muscle mass boost your basic metabolic rate. As I said earlier, your basal metabolic rate contributes approximately sixty percent of the total daily calories you use. Studies have shown that muscle mass, or fat-free mass, is directly related to our basal metabolic rate.[43] This means that resistance training will increase your calorie usage both during and after training."[44]

Steve felt excited. He had enjoyed working out when he was younger.

"That's great news!" he exclaimed. "My doctor told me to lose weight. You mean I just have to start lifting weights and *voilá*, the weight will just come right off?"

"Nope," Rob said, laughing. "If weight loss is your only goal, I would tell you to stick to aerobic exercises. On a time basis, aerobic training will burn more calories than resistance exercises."

Steve's smile disappeared.

"Cheer up, Steve," Rob said, patting Steve on the back. "There are still two more reasons to resistance train aside from weight loss."

"What's that?"

"It's easy to dismiss muscle strength unless we work in a physically demanding profession. But we require muscle strength in all aspects of our life. We lift groceries out of the back of the car, we pick up a child or a pet, and we move boxes in the garage or furniture in the house. We swing a club when we golf or throw a heavy ball down the lane when we bowl.

"As we age, these tasks may become more difficult. Also, daily activities such as moving around the house, getting into a car, or even showering may become difficult. It is easy to overlook our independence until we lose it. Resistance training limits our decline. It allows us to continue to work and play at or near our peak abilities. It allows us to remain self-reliant. As a forty-four-year-old, you may take your functional capacity for granted. But it's not guaranteed."

Steve had grown up near a nursing home. He remembered seeing lots of walkers and wheelchairs.

"For both men and women, but especially women," Rob continued, "osteoporosis is a serious concern. This is the gradual loss of bone density. Resistance training has been shown to maintain bone mineral density and thus delay or maybe even stop osteoporosis from developing."

"I thought only women got osteoporosis."

"It affects more women than men, but it does happen to men, too."

"Finally," Rob concludes, "resistance training can have a positive effect on hormones, including insulin."

Steve's ears perked up. He recalled his doctor telling him that one of his tests showed that he was becoming insulin-resistant.

"Tell me about that," Steve said.

"In one study, older men participating in high-intensity resistance training decreased their homeostasis model assessment of insulin resistance, which is a measurement used to quantify insulin resistance. The participants also showed a ten percent increase in Resting Metabolic Rate and a fifty percent increase in adiponectin levels."[45]

"What is that?"

"Adiponectin is a protein secreted in fat tissue that helps regulate insulin sensitivity and reduce inflammation."[46]

Steve has had enough experience in weight training to understand that diving right into a high-intensity program could be dangerous.

"Are you telling me I have to bench press three hundred pounds for resistance training to help?" Steve asked. "It didn't look like you were lifting a ton of weight, and besides, I wouldn't mind getting Beth involved, and she doesn't know the first thing about weightlifting."

"Heck no," Rob said. "I wouldn't recommend diving into intensive free-weight training. While the best results appear to be from high-intensity exercises, you can still get plenty out of moderate resistance training two or three non-consecutive days a week for a minimum of twenty minutes per session.

"And I wouldn't necessarily recommend free weights. With proper training, free weights are great, but there are many options in choosing a resistance-training regimen. You can do a military-style push-up and pull-up regimen, free weights, or in-home or gym Nautilus training. There are various video workout programs that are effective. If your time is limited or you just hate resistance training, focus your energy on the large muscle groups. Squats or leg presses activate quadriceps, hamstrings, and gluteus muscles. Bench presses and push-ups activate the chest, shoulder, and triceps muscles. And a lat pull-down or pull-up activates the back, shoulder, and biceps muscles.

"Again, even with your past experience you may want to get help or at least go slowly so that you know you're training with the proper technique."

Steve laughed to himself as he recalled all those overzealous knuckle heads lifting more weight than they could handle and injuring themselves.

"Thanks for the refresher and new information, Rob," Steve said. "Beth and I are meeting Matt and Susan for lunch at the diner on sixteenth street if you're interested."

"You mean Susan from the class behind us? I haven't seen her in years. Maybe I'll pop in."

Steve strolled back to the room, thinking, about what Rob had told him. He had thought about taking up weight training again, but it never got past the thinking stage. They had belonged to a gym a few years before, but they never went. He thought about converting the back porch to a workout room, but he wasn't sure what to purchase. He had never considered a personal trainer, but maybe he would look into that as a way to jump-start his training.

When he got back to the room, Beth was gone. She must be at the spa, he thought. He decided to take the opportunity to take a nap before lunch.

Beth returned about a half an hour later. She had enjoyed a one-hour massage that was way too short. She loved her children, and she loved Steve, but she was never alone. The hour with quiet music and a silent but effective massage therapist was blissful.

She heard Steve before she saw him. The television was on, but even it couldn't compete with his snores. She thought it had gotten worse over the past few years as his stomach had grown. A friend told her that Steve might have sleep apnea, an obstruction to breathing while sleeping that is common in overweight and obese people. She used to be able to fall asleep to it, but now she tried to go to bed first or she moved to the sofa.

She looked at the clock. It was 12:15.

She nudged him and said, "Wake up, Steve."

Steve opened his eyes and jumped up. "I'm awake!" he said, looking startled.

"I can't believe you can sleep through that snoring," she said.

"What snoring?" How was your breakfast?"

"It was fun," Beth said. "I ate with Laurie and Ken. She told me that a breakfast with protein and fiber will aid in keeping my energy higher in the morning, and she said that I should look into food intolerances as a remedy for feeling lethargic all day. I'm going to do some research on gluten."

Steve thought about the candy bar and soft drink he had for breakfast.

"What did you do this morning?"

"I ran into Rob. He told me about the benefits of resistance training. He said that I should do some form of training at least twice a week for thirty or more minutes."

Beth smiled as she remembered Steve when he was in shape.

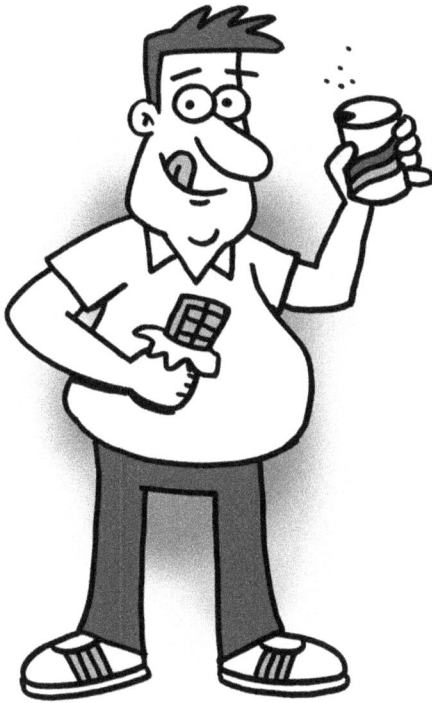

# 7

## FOOD CALORIES AND DENSITY

Steve and Beth got a ride to the diner with Matt. "I'm starving," Steve said. "I had only a candy bar and a soda for breakfast. I could eat a horse."

"What are you doing eating that junk when the doctor told you to eat healthy?" Beth said, clearly annoyed.

"What are you talking about, Beth? I hardly ate anything today.

Matt hesitated to say anything. He had already put in his two cents' worth about NEAT, and he wasn't interested in getting between two fighting spouses. But against his better judgment, he decided to weigh in.

"You do realize that food is not just used to appease our appetite, right?" Matt asked tentatively.

Beth and Steve stared at Matt. Of course they knew that food was more than just an appetite suppresser.

"Doug told me why I eat too much after I skip meals," Steve said.

"And Laurie told me to eat a decent breakfast with protein instead of bread, and she said that I might be gluten-intolerant," Beth added. "And we use the food we eat to produce energy to fuel our bodies."

Matt waited for more, but when they said nothing else, he forged ahead. "That's correct. Food is energy. We need energy to keep our temperature stable, to breath, to eat, and to move. We need energy to keep our heart beating, our muscles contracting, and our organs functioning. We calculate the amount of energy we eat and use it in units called calories."

"Rob was talking to me about calories and resistance exercises earlier," Steve said. "He said something about calories being a unit of energy, but I'm not exactly sure what he meant by that."

"Rob was correct," Matt said. "A calorie is just a unit of energy.[47]   Each gram of protein and carbohydrate contain approximately four calories, and each gram of fat contains approximately nine calories.   To determine the total calories of a food, you multiply each amount of macronutrient in grams by its respective caloric value.[48]"

"That seems simple," Beth said. "If I want to know how many calories I'm eating, I just need a scale and to know the percentage of proteins, carbohydrates, and fats in the food."

"Yes, it seems simple enough," Matt said, "but a large percentage of the weight in food is water.   Also, insoluble fiber, technically a carbohydrate, isn't counted in the caloric calculation. This means you can eat the same amount of food with different numbers of calories."

"Crap!" Beth exclaimed. "I was hoping this would be easy."

"It isn't too difficult," Matt said, "but you need to understand energy density and how different types of foods relate to it.

"Energy density is the number of calories as a percentage of its weight. Foods with high fat content and low water weight are the densest foods. Candy and other sweets with high sugar content tend to be energy dense. Fruits and vegetables contain insoluble fiber and as much as ninety percent water. They are low-density foods."

Steve thought about the candy bar he had eaten that morning.

"Why is energy density important?" Matt asked rhetorically. "When you eat, you don't decide to eat a three-hundred calorie meal. You eat what's on your plate or until you're full- whichever comes first. If you eat a high-density meal, you may easily eat triple the calories in comparison to the same volume of low-density food. At the end of the meal you will have a similar feeling of satiation, but the high-density meal will have greatly increased your caloric intake."

Steve recalled the food he had eaten the night before and Doug's comparison of it to Marcia's meal.

"Also," Doug continued, "dense, high-energy foods are strong predictors of a gain in visceral fat."[49]

"I don't know if you know what visceral fat is," Matt said, looking at Steve. "Visceral body fat is found primarily in the stomach and is a predictor of type-two diabetes, cardiovascular disease, and cancer, after adjusting for body mass index."

There they go again, bringing up my gut, Steve thought. Beth almost seemed relieved. Perhaps this weekend would bring a change. Contrary to popular opinion at the local brewery, a beer belly was not what was missing on Adonis.

"Do you have any examples of high-density and low-density foods?" Beth asked.

"Sure," Matt replied. "One piece of fried chicken at seventy-five grams is two hundred and nineteen calories. An apple is over two hundred and twenty-three grams, yet it only contains a hundred and sixteen calories. Potato chips and doughnuts are other examples of energy-dense foods. Vegetables such as those green leafy things found in the produce section are very low-density foods.

"Go through your pantry and refrigerator and write down the calories per gram of your foods. Food labels are required to list the calories by weight. Energy-dense foods will be high in fat or sugar. Notice the hidden sugars in your canned or boxed foods. What kind of snacks are in your house? Notice how labels show calories per serving. A serving is only a couple of cookies or a few chips. Nobody stops at a couple of cookies!"

Beth and Steve mentally inventoried their cupboards and refrigerator. They were a meat-and-potatoes family, but it was often easier to buy prepared foods. They bought groceries based on coupons or expediency. Neither of them knew the calorie count or energy density of the foods they ate.

They arrived at the restaurant and waited for the host to seat them.

"What type of food do you eat at restaurants?" Matt said. "Small changes to your meal can make a big difference in calories and nutritional value. Every chain restaurant has a list of calories and nutrition online. Make a list of the restaurants you frequent and look up their menus online. If they don't have their nutritional content and calories, find the healthier alternatives by doing some research."

Steve peered at the menu. He had planned to order a double cheeseburger, fries, and a shake. This diner made old-fashioned shakes with whipped cream and a cherry on top. Maybe he'd skip the shake or split it with Beth.

Rob and Susan showed up and they were seated at a round table on the outdoor patio. Susan was a general physician who worked nearby. She had graduated a year after Steve, Rob, and Matt. Beth and Steve had run into her during one of his visits a few years back. Since then, Susan and her husband and children had visited Steve and Beth in Seattle.

Beth was particularly happy to see Susan, who was an amiable person who felt comfortable in her own skin. Besides running her practice and raising two children, she found time to play club volleyball and softball. More importantly, to Beth at least, she didn't talk about football and baseball the whole time.

"How's my favorite city?" Susan said. "Is it still raining all the time?"

Contrary to popular opinion, Seattle does not get a lot of rain. On average it gets around thirty-seven inches a year. But people from the area like the reputation. Seattle was populated enough without the rainophobes adding to it.

"Yep," Beth replied, laughing. "Instead of chains for snow, we carry snorkels on our cars."

"Hi. Matt. , Looks like you've lost some weight since I last saw you," Susan said.

"Thirty pounds!" Matt said, beaming.

"And Steve, you're looking good," Susan lied.

"Thanks," Steve said, holding his stomach. "I'm having Matt ship me the weight he lost so I have extra insulation for my winter coat."

Steve's fat jokes didn't seem as funny under the current circumstances. In hindsight, he wasn't sure whether they were ever funny or if they were just a way of deflecting the issue of his increasing girth. Steve used the opportunity to break the ice about his medical issues.

Steve turned to Susan and said, "I think Beth called you about my blood tests."

Susan nodded.

"I had the opportunity to talk to a cardiologist on the plane coming here. He bluntly explained the numbers. I spoke with Matt about the benefits of NEAT and with Rob about the benefits of resistance training. Matt told us about calories and calorie density as we drove here."

"Sounds like you're getting a good education at your reunion," Susan said.

"Yes, it may be the first time that high school and learning can properly be used in the same sentence for me," Steve joked.

The waiter arrived to take their orders. Steve decided against the double cheese burger and fries with a shake. Instead he ordered a grilled chicken Caesar salad, two slices of wheat bread, and a soft drink.

He smiled to himself at the self-control it took not to order his initial choice.

Susan smiled, too.

"What happened to your regular cheeseburger and fries?" she asked.

"I decided to go with the healthier choice— a salad instead of a cheeseburger, whole wheat toast instead of French fries, and a soft drink instead of a shake."

Susan sighed. She thought about telling him that his choice may have more calories than his initial choice, but she decided to take a different tack.

"Since we're about to eat, perhaps we should talk about how our bodies absorb food," Susan began. "Steve, do you know how your body deals with the food you eat?"

Steve shook his head.

"Digestion is the process of breaking down food into particles small enough for our body to use. The largest sources of particles are called macronutrients—proteins, carbohydrates, and fats. Protein is broken down into amino acids, which are the building blocks of our body. Carbohydrates are broken down into glucose, which is our primary source of energy, and fats are used for storage and additional sources of energy.

"The anticipation of incoming food causes our digestive system to begin secreting enzymes and our insulin levels to rise. This starts a number of reactions.[50] Fats and carbohydrates begin digesting in the mouth, while protein digestion begins in the stomach. Certain dietary fibers work their way through the digestive system, acting as a cleansing system and assisting in digestion."

"Seems like a pretty effective system," Beth said.

"Yes, it is, unless you consistently eat too much." "Eating to excess causes adipocytes, fat cells, to grow in size and number. Your body stores the fat in various places but primarily in the thighs, buttocks, and stomach."

"So I just need to cut down on the amount of fat I eat?" Steve said.

"Unfortunately, it's not just fat that gets stored in your fat cells. The body stores the carbohydrates not needed as glucose or glycogen in your fat cells."

Steve felt confused. The doctor on the plane had explained a little bit about how insulin responds to carbohydrates and helps them get into their proper cells. But Steve couldn't remember his explanation of how the body turned excess glucose into fat.

"Perhaps I should repeat that," Susan said. "That soda you're drinking is full of sugar, or carbohydrates. If your body can't use the sugar, it will store it in your body as fat."

Steve looked at Susan and then his soft drink. This trip was getting worse by the minute.

Susan said, "The foods you eat and drink come in various combinations and types of carbohydrates, fats, and proteins along with micronutrients such as vitamins and minerals. We generally don't think in terms of nutrients when we eat. Our goal is to satisfy our hunger. But from our body's perspective, not all foods are alike. Not only do foods vary in how dense they are in terms of calories per gram, as Matt told you, but they also vary greatly in terms of their nutrient content.

"A simple sandwich can range from a healthy, low-calorie meal to a calorie bomb with limited nutrients. A lean turkey sandwich with lettuce and mustard on whole-grain bread can be a nutritious lunch that contains a number of essential proteins, fats, vitamins, and minerals, all in fewer than three hundred calories. Make a sandwich with salami and mayonnaise with cheese on white bread, and you've eaten well over six hundred empty calories.

"Soft drinks, alcohol, candy, and refined foods are called empty calories because they carry calories that have little nutritional value but count towards your caloric intake. A twelve-ounce soft drink can have over a hundred and fifty calories of sugar. But unless you're an ultra marathoner, your body has little use for that much sugar. Unfortunately, it will do its best to use it all.

"So when was the last time you only drank a twelve-ounce can?" Susan asked Steve, looking at his extra-large cup. "Thirty-two ounces is more the norm—and with free refills. Without blinking, you can add three or four hundred calories a day that have nothing to do but increase your girth."

"I don't drink the soft drink for its nutrient content," Steve said. "I drink it to give me a boost. Anyway, I read that we were supposed to get most of our calories from carbohydrates. Besides, if I'm going to diet, I thought it was fat I needed to avoid."

"I would avoid certain fatty foods because they tend to be high in calories, and certain fats may contribute to cardiovascular problems," Susan said. "However, you wouldn't want to substitute fatty foods for foods high in simple carbohydrates."

"What exactly is a carbohydrate, anyway?" Beth asked.

"Carbohydrates," Susan said, "are foods rich in saccharides or sugars. You will find them in food ranging from fruit, vegetables, and breads to soda, table sugar, and cereal.

"Carbohydrates are broken down in our digestive system into glucose—also called blood sugar—and they are the body's key source of energy. Glucose is used by our nervous system, brain, and red blood cells. When we ingest glucose in the form of carbohydrates, it can end up in one of several places. It can be used for immediate energy, it can be stored as glycogen in the liver, it can be stored in our muscles, or it can be stored in triglycerides as fat. Insulin is the hormone that helps deliver the glucose to these various cells. [51]

Steve's ears perked up at the mention of his pre-diabetic nemesis.

"Insulin opens up muscle and liver cells to accept the increased glucose as glycogen until the amount of glucose in the blood stream decreases," Susan explained. "Excess glucose is converted into fat. Once your blood glucose drops, your insulin levels decrease."

"So what are you saying?" Steve said. "That I should stop eating carbohydrates because they'll just turn into fat?"

"No way!" Susan exclaimed. "I'm saying that not all carbohydrates are the same and that there are some that you should avoid or limit. Perhaps it would be easier if I briefly described the different types of carbohydrates."

Steve said sure, go on.

"Carbohydrates include sugars, starch, and fiber," Susan began. "The simplest carbohydrates are sugars. Refined sugars are those stripped of their nutritional value and added to food to sweeten it. Table sugar is the best known refined sugar. It is a combination of fructose and glucose. You add it to coffee, cookies, and cakes.

"A refined sugar that gets lots of attention is high-fructose corn syrup. This is not actually all fructose but a combination of glucose and fructose.[52] It's used in place of sugar because it's less expensive than sugar. Either simple sugar or high-fructose corn syrup can be found in most processed food. Go to your pantry and read the ingredients on your boxed or canned foods. You will find it difficult to find foods that do not have sugar or high-fructose corn syrup added to them.

"While not all research agrees with it,[53] the evidence linking refined sugars to obesity is substantial. Studies have suggested that fructose consumption tends to increase visceral body fat, while glucose consumption favors subcutaneous fat.[54] Fructose also has a number of other harmful effects. It tends to turn to fat more quickly than glucose; it increases the concentration of small LDL cholesterol, the bad cholesterol; and it does not require insulin for a key part of its metabolism, thus promoting insulin resistance.[55] Because of the way refined sugars are digested, their calorie content and their dearth of nutritional value, when looking to reduce calories, refined sugars should be at the top of the list."

"Do you mean to tell me that Steve's breakfast of a soft drink and a candy bar or donuts is not healthy?" Beth said with a smile.

"At least he's not skipping breakfast," Susan said. "But yes, I would say he's eating about four hundred empty calories to start his day."

"What the heck are you talking about empty?" Steve replied. "My last meal had peanuts in it. Airline food is nutritious, isn't it?"

They all laugh.

"I'm sure one of the food groups was in your breakfast," Rob said, punching Steve's arm.

Susan smiled. "Another form of sugar is polyols, also called sugar alcohol," she said. "Don't get excited, Steve, it's not actually an alcohol."

Steve smiled, but he was still thinking about his lost breakfasts.

"Sugar alcohols are carbohydrates found in a variety of fruits and vegetables, and they're also manufactured from sugar. The number of calories in sugar alcohols varies but on average is about two point four calories per gram or about sixty percent of the calories of regular sugar. They are also converted to glucose more slowly than sugar, which reduces their effect on insulin. Because they have a lower caloric count than sugar and have less effect on insulin, they are often used as an additive with artificial sweeteners.

"However, sugar alcohols are not as sweet as sugar. Therefore, it takes more sugar alcohol to equal the same taste as sugar. To achieve the same taste, more sugar alcohol is added, thus reducing the dietary benefits. Also, sugar alcohol is not fully absorbed by the small intestine. This can cause some bloating and diarrhea if eaten in excess."

"If sugar and sugar alcohols are simple carbohydrates, what is an example of an unsimple carbohydrate?" Steve asked.

"Starch is a complex carbohydrate made up of glucose molecules," Susan said. "It is the most common carbohydrate found in foods. Potatoes, rice, beans, lentils, corn, and grains such as wheat, barley, oats, and rice contain starch. Starches, primarily wheat starch, are often added to foods in order to thicken them. Because of its prevalence and cost, wheat is the major source of starch in the United States, and it can be a nutritious source of calories.

"Unrefined wheat products contain dietary fiber in addition to the starch. The fiber increases the digestive process of the wheat and is beneficial to the digestive tract. However, wheat is often stripped of its fiber and any other nutrients. And sugar may be added to increase palatability. If you aren't careful, ultimately you may be eating a calorie-rich, nutrient-free food."

"So instead of white toast for breakfast, I should have whole wheat toast?" said Matt, who was a big bread eater.

"No," Susan replied. "Look for whole grain bread. Whole wheat bread often has the same nutrient content as white bread."

"You mentioned dietary fiber," Steve said. "You're not suggesting I start eating bran, are you?"

"You may want to start eating bran, Steve. Dietary fiber is a complex carbohydrate that is resistant to digestion. Fiber is found in fruits, vegetables, whole grains, oats, wheat bran, and nuts.[56] Dietary fiber may play a role in the prevention of diabetes. Fiber slows the absorption of food in the digestive system so that fat and carbohydrates remain there longer, aiding their digestion. Fiber also plays a role in satiety, which increases the amount of time between meals and reduces the amount of food eaten in the next meal. Also, fiber improves bowel function, increases insulin sensitivity, and decreases proteins active during inflammation.[57]

"However," Susan said, "overeating fiber without drinking plenty of water can reduce the absorption of proteins, vitamins, and minerals."

"Sugars, starch, and fiber," Steve said. "Avoid sugars, but eat foods that break down to glucose and part of sugar. This seems very complicated."

"Let's make it simpler," Susan said, "and look at the lunch you just ate."

Steve looked at his empty plate and cringed.

"You had a grilled chicken Caesar salad," Susan said.

"Yes, I went with a healthy choice instead of my normal double cheeseburger."

"You aren't alone when you think that you're eating healthy when you eat a salad," Susan said. "While salads can be very nutritious, with a few additions they can be unhealthy calorie bombs. You, Steve, had a calorie bomb."

"Don't mince words, Susan," Steve said.

"On the upside, it had romaine lettuce. This leafy vegetable is a good source of vitamins, minerals, and fiber. It has greater nutritional value than iceberg lettuce, which is a common lettuce found in most salads. You really cannot go wrong with any leafy green vegetable like broccoli, kale, and spinach because they are excellent sources of fiber, vitamins, minerals, and other nutrients.

"Chicken can be an excellent source of protein. Unfortunately, the restaurant marinated it in ingredients that included sugar, which increases the carbohydrate and calorie content. I would look for grilled, baked, or roasted chicken that is not breaded. I would also try to find free-range, hormone-free chicken.

"The salad dressing also contains sugar, among other ingredients. And it has croutons, which are just breads stripped of their nutritional content. My guess is that your salad had close to seven hundred calories.

"The wheat bread may have been enriched with vitamins, but wheat bread should not be confused with whole grain bread. Wheat bread has been processed in a way that strips it of many of its nutrients and fiber content. While your body processes whole grain breads slowly as it goes through the digestive system, wheat and white breads are processed more quickly, causing a spike in insulin and thus contributing to your potential insulin resistance. With the butter added to it, you had an additional hundred and sixty calories.

"Finally, there's your soft drink. At three dollars a drink, free refills are an easy added value item for the restaurant. But they also increase the huge number of calories consumed. You had one refill of your large glass. Subtracting the ice in your drink, I'm going to guess you had well over twenty ounces of that soft drink. That means you had over two hundred calories in your drink and over fifty grams of sugar. In one sitting you exceeded the recommended daily allowance of sugar by ten grams. And that's not including the sugar in your meal."

"Wow, that's over a thousand calories!" Beth said.

"That right," Susan said. "And with the exception of the lettuce and the chicken, the nutritional content of the meal was negligible."

"Is a thousand calories a lot?" Steve asked.

"Yes, it's a lot. But it's the type of calories that concerns me as much as the number of calories. Foods high in simple carbohydrates such as soft drinks, refined breads and even juices spike your insulin, because it needs to respond to the influx of sugar and other simple carbohydrates."

"Juices?" Rob said.

"Fruits are an excellent source of vitamins and minerals, but fruits are high in fiber, which slows down their digestion. Fruit juices are often stripped of the fruit's fiber, and they can have sugar added to them. Check the ingredients on the fruit juices. You will find that they can have as many calories and sugar as the equivalent size soft drink."

"I have lots of fruit juices at home for me and my children," Rob said.

"They aren't completely worthless, because they may have some vitamins in them, but I would feed them the fruit and give them water to drink instead."

I've heard of something called the glycemic index," Matt said. "Is that related to what you're talking about?"

"The glycemic index is a measure of the increase in glucose in the blood system after eating carbohydrates," Susan explained. "Because of the relationship between glucose, insulin, and Metabolic Syndrome, the speed that carbohydrates are broken down into glucose as they are digested plays an import role in our health. The glycemic index measures how quickly your glucose or blood sugar rises when you eat fifty grams of a food containing carbohydrates. The higher the number, the greater the impact on blood sugar and the greater the number." [58]

"So if a food has a high glycemic index, Steve should avoid it so he doesn't spike his insulin?" Beth asked.

"I wish it was that simple. Unfortunately, we don't eat food in fifty gram portions. Since the amount of carbohydrates varies in different food servings, you can eat a food with a high glycemic index that has less glucose response when compared to a food with a lower glycemic index that has high carbohydrate content. The glycemic load was designed with this in mind. Glycemic load is the glycemic index multiplied by the grams of carbohydrates in the food and then divided by one hundred.

"Diets with high glycemic loads have been positively associated with elevated cholesterol and triglyceride levels as well as an elevated risk of coronary heart disease.[59] I'm a little skeptical about the glycemic index because there are variations in the testing results, and it doesn't take into account how foods with a high glycemic index respond when eaten with other foods. But it's another resource in your quest for healthy foods."

"Well, this sucks," Steve said. "I eat what I think of as a healthy meal, and you tell me it was a nutrition nightmare. My soft drinks are liquid calories that want to rush to my gut. I drink light beer so at least that can't be too bad. But what the hell is next? Are you going to tell me that watching baseball causes cancer?"

Susan laughed. "Who knows, it seems like everything else does. What I will say is that when I have patients who need to drop some weight, my first piece of advice is 'don't drink your calories.' My second piece of advice is to tell them to avoid or at least reduce their intake of refined foods, packaged foods, and sugars."

"By don't drink your calories, are you including light beer?" Steve asked.

"Watch out, Susan," Beth said, "you're talking about one of Steve's food groups."

"Yes, beer is included," Susan replied. "I'm not saying that you have to stop drinking alcohol to be healthy. Recent studies have promoted the benefits of drinking in moderation. Red wines contain resveratrol, an antioxidant. Drinking alcohol in moderation has shown its ability to reduce the risk of diabetes, strokes, and heart disease. The risk of dementia in older adults was lowered with the consumption of one to six drinks a week. [60]

"While small levels of alcohol may be beneficial, alcohol has a number of health risks. Alcohol has been linked to sleep disorders, depression, and suicide. Entire industries have grown around alcohol abuse. Aside from the extra calories you're drinking when you have a beer, it's worth understanding how alcohol works in our body.

"Alcohol does not require digestion to enter the bloodstream. It enters through the stomach and small intestine. The liver, acting as garbage man, is the primary organ charged with cleaning out the effects of alcohol. As such, over time it takes the most abuse.[61]

"Alcohol intake can lead to malnutrition, either by using the alcohol calories in place of nutritional calories or by the way alcohol interferes with metabolism, including the absorption of proteins and vitamins. Malnutrition can lead to liver disease separately from the effects of alcohol on the liver. It may interfere with the digestion of essential amino acids, including albumin, which is used to maintain normal blood volume. Alcohol also makes it more difficult to absorb essential vitamins such as vitamin $B_1$, which can cause a thiamine deficiency. Excessive alcohol consumption can lead to liver diseases from fatty liver to fibrosis and ultimately cirrhosis. Cirrhosis leads to death within four years for fifty percent of the people who get it. [62]

"Besides that, alcoholic beverages contain significant amounts of empty calories. Drink two or three beers a night—and yes, Steve, even light beers—and you can add three hundred to five hundred calories to your daily intake. Mixed drinks may not be much better. Alcoholic drinks don't add nutritional value and are not a substitute for a real meal, but they add to food intake and are great contributors to weight gain."

Susan took a breath. The food had come, but she hadn't been able to eat. They finished their meals and talked about the reunion, their families, and jobs. Susan's practice was busy with both real and imagined health issues. Beth mentioned her conversation with Laurie, and they decided to meet later that day and talk about it.

Steve was normally on stage at gatherings, but the late night and large lunch made him tired. Besides, he had a lot to think about.

They said their good-byes, and Matt, Beth, and Steve headed back to the hotel. Before they went to their respective rooms, Matt and Steve agreed to go hiking later that afternoon.

"Well, that lunch sucked," Steve said.

"What are you talking about?" Beth said. "I thought it was great. Matt told us to be aware of energy-dense foods such as those with high fat content or simple carbohydrates and how they can increase caloric content over similar amounts of low-dense foods such as fruits and vegetables. Susan told us how simple carbohydrates such as sugars and refined breads spike your insulin and turn into fat."

"She also said that we should eat fruits, vegetables, and whole grains instead of simple carbohydrates, because they contain fiber that aids in digestion, they're digested more slowly, and they're high in nutrients," Steve said.

"And don't forget her suggestion to avoid or limit drinking your calories with soft drinks, sugared juices, and alcohol," Beth added.

Steve scowled at his wife. "Thanks for reminding me, Beth."

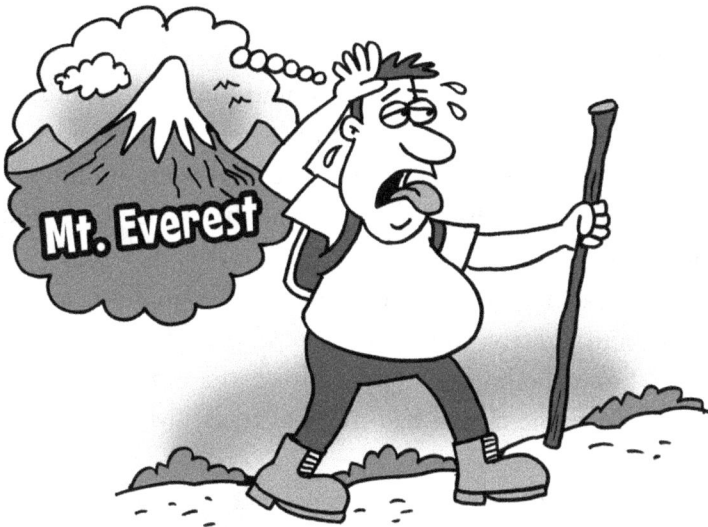

# 8

## ENDURANCE TRAINING

Steve slept for two hours. He and Beth had come back and gone to the lazy river pool to relax. The weather was a little cold for the locals but perfect for them. Steve was going to order a drink but decided against it. He had agreed to the stupid hike with Matt, and he knew it would be difficult enough without alcohol. Beth ordered a Strawberry Daiquiri.

The drink would have been wasted on Steve. Within fifteen minutes of lying down, he was out cold.

Cold water on his face startled Steve awake. It was Matt and Rob.

"What the heck are you guys doing?" Steve said, feeling annoyed.

"Sorry," Matt said. "We thought you were stuck in a meditative state in a quest to find your inner Buddha and needed the jolt."

"Besides, you're late," Rob said. "We were supposed to meet in the back of the resort fifteen minutes ago. You didn't want us to go without you, did you?"

He did want them to go without him, but he didn't say it.

"Let me grab my shoes on our way," Steve said. "I'm heading out, Beth. Call for help if I'm not back in twenty minutes."

Beth waved him off with a laugh. "You think you'll last that long, old man?" Rob said.

Steve chuckled, but the irony of the question wasn't wasted on Beth or him. Lately, twenty minutes would set some type of record.

From the hotel they could hike to a mountain preserve. Set in the middle of the city, it had miles of trails. Many hikers and runners spent hours there.

Steve's time frame was more like minutes than hours. In his twenties he had hiked in the Cascades in Washington and Oregon. He had endurance and strength, so an all-day hike wasn't intimidating. Twenty years later, he stared up at the small mountain and sighed.

"How far do you want to go?" asked Matt.

"You saw me last night, Matt," Steve replied. "I just want to hike enough to work off my lunch."

Matt laughed. "Unless you're an ultra-marathon runner, triathlete, or a Tour de France rider, or you spend an extraordinary amount of time performing physical activity, you can't out-exercise excessive overeating. Depending on your weight, a mile of running will burn approximately a hundred and ten calories. You can wipe out the caloric benefits of a ten-mile run with one supersize meal."[63]

"Of course the calories burned during exercise can help you lose weight," Rob said. "You have to burn thirty-five hundred more calories than you eat and drink to lose a pound. If you exercised and ate the same, you would begin to lose weight. But most people eat more calories as a reward for exercise."

Steve felt disappointed. What had he gotten himself into?

"Then why bother hiking?" Steve asked, feeling exasperated.

"Exercise doesn't just burn calories," Matt said. "It has other physiological benefits, including increased basal metabolic rate and a reduction in Metabolic Syndrome symptoms. Being physically fit is associated with reduced risk of cardiovascular disease and cancer. It also lessens the risk of mortality once you have cancer or cardiovascular disease.[64] And it can boost your immune system. It has also been shown to increase insulin sensitivity and reduce inflammation."[65]

"It can improve motor coordination and flexibility, too," said Rob, "and it lowers the risk of arthritis in older adults.[66] Exercise can aid in increased bone density and lower the incidence of bone fractures. As we age we may have ambulatory difficulties and thus an increased risk of disability."

Steve thought about his parents. When you're young you think of your parents as all-knowing, all-powerful immortal beings who will always be there. As teenagers you thought of them as morons who would never go away. As a parent you realize just how much they cared. But as your parents grow old, you begin to recognize their frailties. You understand that it may be you taking care of them. You see the importance of health from a different angle.

Steve's mom had been overweight for most of his life. She had trouble walking, so she used a motorized cart to transport herself whenever she had to go any distance. He didn't know if her weight caused her difficulties. She claimed she had bad hips and knees. He does know that if it's something he can prevent, he will do his best to try.

"Finally, exercise has a number of psychological benefits," Rob said. "You will increase your sense of well-being. You will reduce stress and lower the likelihood of depression or anxiety disorders.

"So don't look so disappointed, Steve," Rob said.

Steve managed a smile. They had been hiking for only ten minutes, and he could feel the effects in his lungs. Neither Matt nor Rob was winded.

"After talking to Rob at the gym, I was thinking about just doing some weightlifting for my exercise," Steve said. "Now you guys are telling me I need to run, too!"

"I don't think you have to run," Matt said. "In fact, at your weight, I would recommend a different form of aerobic exercise.

Running may be hard on your joints until you reduce your weight. I would recommend some other form of endurance training."[67]

Steve would have tackled Matt if he hadn't been so tired.

"What do you mean by endurance training?" Steve asked.

"Endurance training is exercise designed to increase aerobic fitness," Matt replied. "Since aerobic exercises like running, swimming, and cycling require oxygen to sustain effort over a period of time, aerobic fitness is gauged by the amount of oxygen a person can take in and use at or near total exertion, called $VO_2$ max. Like muscle mass, $VO_2$ max declines as we age. And also like muscle mass, exercise, specifically endurance exercise, increases $VO_2$ max. Aside from being able to hike past your neighbor without gasping for air, aerobic fitness has a strong correlation with reduced Metabolic Syndrome factors." [68]

Steve thought that his $VO_2$ max must be pretty low by now. Matt and Rob told him that they were only going on a short hike. It felt like an eternity at this point.

"You listening, Steve?" Rob asked as he walked backward in front of him, just out of reach.

Steve didn't have the breath to tell him where to go.

"This looks like a good place to stop," Matt said. He took out a water bottle and drank some.

They could see the west Phoenix valley from this height. For the geometrically challenged, Phoenix is a dream city. It is one large grid, with Central Avenue bisecting the east and west sides of it. If they were a little higher, they could see the houses where they grew up a few miles west. Steve shook the thought of those being simpler times as something his dad would say.

"Tell me about the research on Metabolic Syndrome and endurance exercises," Steve said.

"Yes, your vastness," Matt said, bowing to him. "Researchers studied a group of overweight, sedentary men and women who showed signs of Metabolic Syndrome. The researchers had them walk the equivalent of twelve miles a week. The participants showed an increase in $VO_2$ max and time to exhaustion, two indicators of reduced cardiovascular disease. Another group participating in the same study jogged or ran twenty miles. They showed an even greater increase in calories used and VO$_2$ max."[69] [70]

"Endurance training alters how our bodies use up fat and carbohydrates," Rob explained. "As we become more efficient at training, our body begins to use up fat over carbohydrates as its source of energy.[71],[72] It may also increase your HDL cholesterol—the good cholesterol—and lower LDL cholesterol—the bad cholesterol.[73]"

When they headed back, Steve took each step carefully. He was still shaky from the hike up, and at 235 pounds, going downhill was scarier than going uphill.

"Do I need to breathe as hard as I am on this climb?" Steve asked. "I was beginning to think you guys were going to have to drag my butt back to the hotel."

"Nah, we would've left you out here," Rob said. "You're mug would have decorated the opening of some coyote's den."

"I was thinking he would be splayed out in some cave as a cougar's rug," Matt said.

"I'll kick both your butts when I catch my breath," Steve said.

"Where were we?" Rob asked, laughing.

"I was asking if I have to breathe like a twelve-year-old girl at a boy-band concert," Steve said.

"Most aerobic training focuses on moderate intensities over extended periods of time," Matt said. "However, there is evidence that high-intensity, intermittent exercise may be more effective at reducing body fat and improving other Metabolic Syndrome factors. High-intensity intermittent training is exercise for short periods of maximum effort followed by periods of rest. The maximum effort can be as short as six seconds and as long as four minutes. The rest period can range from twelve seconds to more than four minutes.[74]

"A review of this type of training found that participants showed a decline in body fat, including abdominal fat, weight loss, and an increase in insulin sensitivity.[75] The upside of high-intensity, intermittent training is that it requires less time than standard endurance training. The training sessions lasted as little as twenty minutes."

"But I think high-intensity exercise may be too difficult for people when they're starting out," Rob said. "In fact, I think high-intensity training may be too difficult to sustain long-term. If you're thinking of taking up some form of aerobic training, Steve, be cautious before jumping into an intense regimen. You will feel great for a while, but it will be easy to over-train. I think you're better off doing a lower-intensity exercise that you will enjoy long-term."

"There's only one problem with all this talk about aerobic exercise," Steve said. "I hate running."

Rob laughed. "Well, then don't run. You have tons of options when it comes to aerobic training. You can swim, bike, join an aerobics class, row, hop on an elliptical machine. For people new to training or if you have difficulty doing any level of exercise, I would start with water aerobics. Water makes you buoyant and reduces the pressure on your joints. I think it's an option that many people overlook when they start an endurance training program.

"You can also purchase an exercise video, or join a soccer team or ice hockey team," Matt said.

"Just keep in mind, the first few weeks of any new endurance training will be difficult," Matt added. "You are awakening sleeping muscles. They will not be happy. You will tire quickly, and you will feel a little tired after you're finished and maybe the next day, too."

Rob threw his arm across Steve's shoulders as they re-entered the resort. "You will often see people choose an event like a 5k run or a marathon as motivation to exercise. If finding some event to compete gets you out the door, go for it. However, once the event is finished, pat yourself on the back and get back on the road or in the pool or on the bike. Don't view it as if you conquered Mount Everest. Look at it as a small part of a lifelong journey."

Steve laughed. For him, they had just climbed Mount Everest.

Steve found Beth still reading by the pool. It seemed like an eternity, but it was less than an hour from the time he had left. He talked to Beth about his conversation with Rob and Matt. He told her that he was thinking about getting his mountain bike out of the garage and taking up riding again. Beth wondered how long it had been since that bike saw asphalt.

They spent the next hour reading by the pool before Beth had to go. She was meeting Susan in the hotel lounge. Steve was invited, but he decided to let them have time to themselves. Besides, he hadn't seen a sports update in more than six hours. As a PAC-Ten guy, most of the games he cared about were played at night. But he still liked watching football even if it wasn't his team.

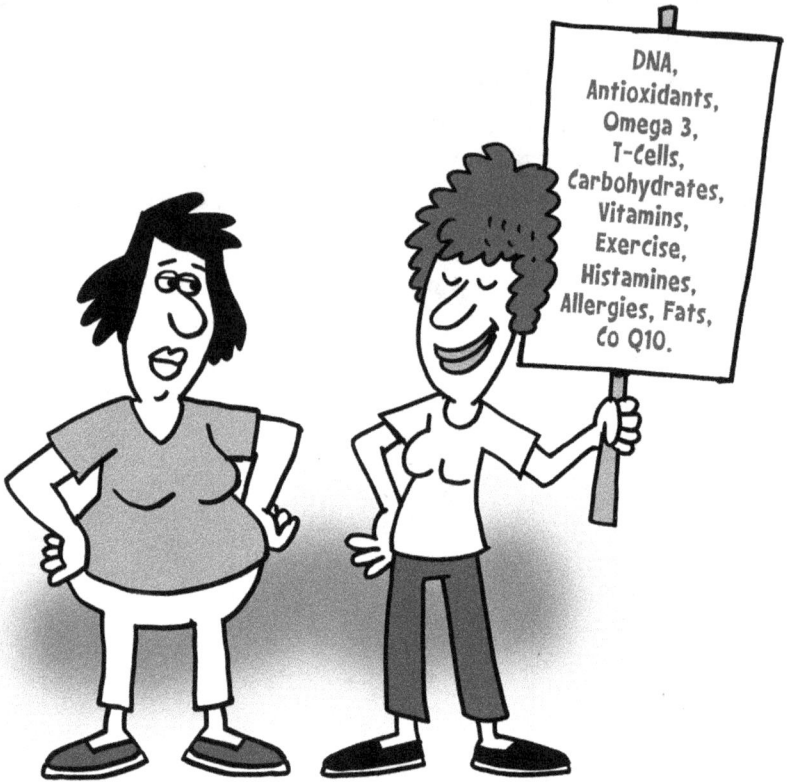

DNA, Antioxidants, Omega 3, T-Cells, Carbohydrates, Vitamins, Exercise, Histamines, Allergies, Fats, Co Q10.

# 9

# THE IMMUNE SYSTEM AND OXIDATIVE STRESS

Beth looked forward to meeting with Susan. Saturday night was sure to be a repeat of the night before only with more people. It would be nice to talk to someone without a bunch of drunks stumbling around. Besides, she enjoyed Susan's company. She found many of the doctors to be aloof. But Susan was as comfortable talking about her teenage daughters as she was her medical practice. Steve usually bowed out of these talks. He said that when two women got together he could never understand them. He said it seemed as if we spoke a different language. Beth agreed. Women call it English, she thought.

The lounge was in the front of the hotel. Beth and Susan sat at a table on the front patio. It was five in the afternoon, and the place was quiet. Susan worked one Saturday a month at a clinic in central Phoenix. She lived in north Phoenix, so the resort was located on her way home.

"How was your afternoon?" Susan asked.

"It was fantastic," said Beth. "I love my kids, but it's nice to have a quiet day all to myself."

Susan sighed. "I wish I knew what you meant. My girls have ten things going on at once. Bill and I are glorified chauffeurs. But with my eldest turning sixteen in two months, I think my taxi days are numbered."

"I say that it's nice to have a quiet day, but believe me, it goes quickly," Beth said. "My oldest daughter is twenty-three. It seems like I was changing her diapers yesterday. Zack will be driving in a year, which means he'll be basically gone." Beth was silent for a while.

"See what you did? You made me miss the little brats."

The conversation wound around the children and their careers. Beth and Susan had managed to successfully navigate both, though Beth worried about Sara and her tendency to hide in her room.

"Who else have you seen at the reunion?" Susan said.

"We saw Marcia and Ivan last night. Marcia looked good. It looks like her gastric bypass surgery was a success. But Ivan looked terrible."

"I'm happy for Marcia. I not a fan of surgery if it's not absolutely necessary; but it's nice to hear that it worked for her."

"Oh, and I saw Laurie last night and this morning. She told me that she's now gluten-free."

Susan cocked her head. "There is more and more research being done on the foods we eat and our bodies' response to them. I have plenty of patients who seem to be chronically ill. We tend to point to the outside environment, but it could be certain foods are weakening our immune system and making us more susceptible to viruses and bacteria."

"Aside from being annoyed when I get a cold, I know very little about how my immune system works," Beth said.

"I like to view our immune system as an army," Susan said. "Whenever you get sick or cut yourself or have an allergy, your immune system responds. Its job is to seek out foreign invaders, destroy them, and flush them out of your body. The primary soldiers in this army are white blood cells. The foreign invader is called a pathogen. It can come from infection, bacteria, internal hemorrhage, cuts in the skin, or even an internal rupture of a cell.

"Histamines—the annoying chemical that makes your nose run and your eyes water when you have an allergy—are some of the first responders to a foreign invader. They enlarge the capillaries around the invasion, which allows the white blood cells to quickly reach the affected site. Neutrophils, the most common white blood cells, are the first to the site, where they ingest some of the foreign cells.

"Also attracted to the area are monocytes, which reach the site and divide into macrophages and dentrites. Macrophages recognize the pathogens and engulf them and produce an antigen. The antigen is recognized by T-cells. The T-cells secrete a chemical that warns natural killer cells. These cells, as you would expect, kill the pathogens or cells infected by the pathogens.

"In addition to natural killer cells, T-cell helpers call on B-cells to aid in the fight. B-cells generate antibodies that proliferate in the bloodstream and recognize the specific antigen part of the pathogen. The antibodies bind to the antigen and make their way to the macrophage, where they are ingested and destroyed. Other B-cells develop a code that will recognize the antigen if it ever has the temerity to resurface.

"Have you ever wondered about what an allergic reaction really is?"

Beth nodded her head.

"An allergic reaction is a response by your immune system to a foreign invader. Red eyes and congestion are the histamines responding to pollen being inhaled or a reaction to certain foods."

"What a great system," Beth said. "So we have cells built to recognize a foreign invader and surround it and send out a bugle call to its comrades, who in turn break it down and send it back out of your body?"

"That's right. And as part of your immune response, capillaries open up to allow these additional cells to work their magic. Also, the immune system manufactures B-cells that develop a code for that particular antigen so that if the antigen returns, it is quickly destroyed."

"That's really amazing," Beth said.

"Of course the immune system isn't perfect. The immune cells may attack healthy cells in a mistaken response to a perceived attack. The pathogens that invade may be small, but they aren't stupid. Some pathogens mimic healthy cells and freely roam your body, doing damage. The immune system responds to any cell damage, including damage caused by reactive oxidative stress."

"What the heck is that?"

"Reactive oxidative stress is a result of our body's failure to clean up harmful atoms or molecules. These molecules are referred to as free radicals. These molecules target and harm proteins, fats, carbohydrates, and DNA cells.[76] When we're young our body creates enzymes and antioxidants that remove the free radicals. Unfortunately, as we age we have fewer antioxidants, so the free radicals begin to damage our cells and our immune system.

"If we don't increase antioxidants or decrease the free radicals, we end up with chronic inflammation."

"Why is that a problem?"

"It means your body is in continuous fight mode."

"Wouldn't I notice if my body was always battling these free radicals?"

"Not necessarily. I equate it to a slow loss of hearing. If you lost half of your ability to hear overnight, you'd panic and go see a doctor immediately. But if you lost half of your ability to hear over a twenty-year period, you may not even notice it."

"I think Steve is suffering from hearing loss. I always have to repeat myself."

"I think that's a defect in all men, Beth," Susan replied with a laugh.

"The subtle deterioration that you can get with hearing loss is the same with chronic inflammation," Susan continued. "When you get a cold, you know immediately that your immune system has been compromised. Chronic inflammation weakens your immune system over time. It makes you more tired, it tends to leave people with a nonspecific sense of malaise, and it lends itself to more illnesses.

"I would be happy to talk to Steve about this because oxidative stress has been implicated in Metabolic Syndrome[77] and sarcopenia, or muscle loss, as we age.[78] [79] People with Metabolic Syndrome have lower amounts of vitamin C and E and antioxidants."

"So you're saying that a person in Steve's position has fewer antioxidants than a person who does not have Metabolic Syndrome symptoms and they are also less likely to eat the foods that will increase their antioxidants?"

"Yes, that's right."

"It appears as if oxidative stress and inflammation are strongly related to each other," Beth said. "Does that mean that if I reduce the amount of oxidative stress in my system, I will reduce the inflammation?"

"Right again. It turns out that the type of foods we eat and exercise both play a role in diminishing free radicals and inflammation."[80, 81]

Beth had been taking notes as Susan spoke. She thought about the food they ate. They had vegetables for dinner occasionally. But they rarely ate fruit, and she doubted that Steve ate a healthy meal at lunch.

"I can just e-mail you this information, Beth."

Beth hesitated to reply. Despite being computer-savvy, she still found herself using pen and paper whenever she wanted to put her thoughts down.

"The list of foods that have antioxidant effects are numerous but revolve around fruits and vegetables. Eating a diet of fish, vegetables, fruits, and whole grains will increase the antioxidants and reduce inflammation and free radicals. Drinking orange juice with a high-fat, high-carbohydrate meal may neutralize the pro-inflammatory effects of the meal. Also, a high-fiber and high-fruit meal does not induce oxidative or inflammatory stress when compared to an equivalent high-fat, high-carbohydrate meal.[82]

"There are also a number of other reasons to eat more fruits and vegetables," Susan said. "Certain fruits and vegetables contain flavenoids and resveratrol, which both help remove antioxidants."

"What are flavenoids and resveratrol?"

Flavenoids[83] are the byproduct of certain plants that also have antioxidant attributes. Eating foods high in flavenoids has been shown to reduce obesity. [84] Foods containing high flavenoid content of some sort include onions, leeks, tea—brewed and nondecaffeinated have the highest flavenoid content—apples, pears, chocolate, blueberries, tofu, cranberry juice, and sweet potatoes.[85]

"Resveratrol, primarily found in red grapes, cocoa powder, mulberries, blackberries, and peanuts, suppresses reactive oxygen species. Vegetables with antioxidants include beans—pinto beans and red and black beans—and russet potatoes, and fruits with antioxidants include blueberries, raspberries, cranberries, plums, apples, cherries, prunes, and pecans.[86]

"Other foods can also affect antioxidants and inflammation. Curcumin, a product of turmeric, and Indian spice are anti-inflammatory. Fish and fish oil with Omega-3 fatty acids has anti-inflammatory effects."[87]

"That's an extensive list," Beth said.

"I know. Notice they almost all revolve around the produce section of the grocery store. Most people spend a majority of their time and money in the boxed and canned food sections of the store."

"But boxed and canned foods store well, and they're easy to make," Beth said defensively. "Produce goes bad if it's not eaten within a few days."

"There are ways to store produce so that it will last longer," Susan said. "Maybe you can go online and find out which fruits and vegetables last a little longer."

"Finally," Susan said, "you should know about coenzyme $Q_{10}$, or Co $Q_{10}$, supplementation, which may have a number of benefits. It has been shown to reduce the risk of heart failure and to lower blood pressure in patients suffering from hypertension. It may also improve insulin resistance."[88]

They sat there silently for a couple of minutes, while Beth scribbled notes. Susan thought about how different her practice would be without chronic illnesses. The 80/20 rule worked in medicine. She spent eighty percent of her time with twenty percent of her patients. She was quite capable of prescribing antibiotics and other prescription drugs to these patients, but she couldn't help but think that a lifestyle change would be the best remedy. But the health care system didn't encourage that. Small or no co-payments had made it easier to use the doctor as a substitute for a healthier lifestyle.

"Oh, and don't forget about exercise," Susan said. "Physical activity also reduces the inflammatory response."[89]

"I'm glad to hear that. Steve and I used to be very active, but we let kids and work get in the way. It would be great if we could start exercising again. I always felt better when I was in shape."

Susan said she had to be home soon. They said good-bye and promised to keep in touch. Susan said she would e-mail Beth the information on inflammation and antioxidants.

Beth walked back to the casita. Susan had plenty of information that might help Steve, so she was looking forward to passing it along to him. But she thought about her own health issues, too. She had signs of perimenopause, including missed periods, difficulty sleeping, fatigue, and moodiness. She was planning to see a hormone specialist. After speaking with Laurie and Susan, she thought maybe these problems were related to her diet.

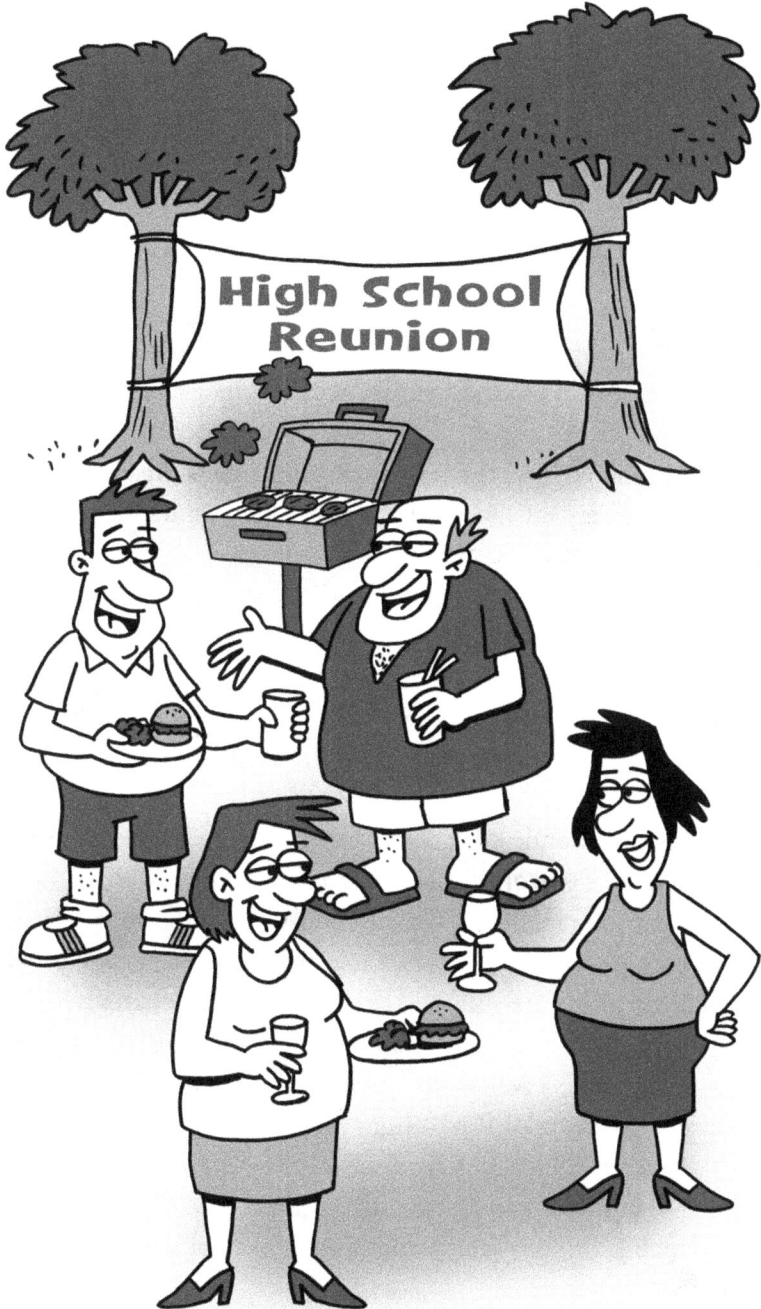

# 10

## FATS AND PROTEINS

The reunion committee had set up a barbeque area at the western-style restaurant at the resort. It had floors covered with sod and an outdoor barbecue pit. Country music twanged through the restaurant. The staff wore jeans and checkered red-and-blue button-down, cowboy-style shirts. The bar, made up as a nineteenth-century saloon, was located a few steps below the restaurant floor.

To complete the country-western motif, an abandoned corral sat behind the restaurant. The reunion attendees sat in the back, next to the corral. Wendy, the post-high school class organizer, had planned the event. Everyone wore a name tag so they could identify their fellow classmates, because the passage of time was not always kind.

Each reunion member could enjoy a meal with a salad, entrée, two sides, and dessert as part of their pre-paid plan. This was not the place to start his weight-loss program, Steve thought. He wore cowboy boots and beat-up old jeans for the occasion. Beth wore a denim skirt and a white embroidered sleeveless shirt. If a square dance broke out, they would be ready.

Steve wandered around, checking out the decorations the organizers had put on display. An old letterman's jacket hung from a fence post. A table held the yearbooks from the four years they had attended high school. But the table that grabbed Steve's attention had six pictures of old classmates. They were the classmates who had passed away since graduation. A couple of them had died when they took their own life. Five of the pictures he recognized from the prior reunion. A picture of Ron caught Steve's eye.

"Heart attack," Doug said, startling Steve.

"He was at our last reunion," Steve said, feeling stunned. "He was dancing on the tables and singing karaoke without the karaoke machine."

"Yeah, well here's to Ron," Doug said, lifting his glass. "Life is short. We just don't always know how short it is."

They touched glasses. Yes, life is short, he thought. What a way to start the evening, he thought.

Steve and Beth sat with Charlene and Mike, along with Wendy and her husband, Allan. Wendy was a housewife with three growing boys who kept her running. Allan was a lobbyist who worked near the state capital.

Allan was fastidious about his health. Before joining a lobbying firm, he was a registered dietician at a local nursing home. He still kept up with health issues as a hobby.

Wendy didn't share Allan's love for all that is healthy. She was a serial dieter. Run into her on the right day, and she would be thin, exercising, eating healthy foods, and preaching about her newfound ways. A few months later, and you would find her on the couch, eating a pork belly sandwich with chips and topping off her meal with an ice cream chaser. At the reunion, Wendy was her gluttonous self.

Steve remembered Charlene as a heavy girl. He had gone to school with her from third grade until they graduated from high school. He had a limited memory of her because they had run in different crowds. She was not heavy anymore. He wouldn't call her skinny, but she was on the lighter side of average.

"I'm starving, where's our waitress?" Mike hollered. At six-three and 225 pounds, Mike was a big guy with a big appetite.

Steve nodded in agreement. He was famished. He loved steak and potatoes. He was extra excited because he could eat a little extra since he had hiked that afternoon. As soon as he thought this he remembered Rob's saying that he could not out-exercise his eating. He decided not to go overboard.

Steve ordered a salad with ranch dressing, a steak with béarnaise sauce, garlic mashed potatoes, and corn-on-the cob. He ate potatoes, corn, and a salad. It was a vegetable medley, so it must be healthy, he thought. Besides, the choices on the menu were limited.

About forty people showed up for the dinner. He was disappointed that a couple of his old running buddies didn't make it, but he could find fun in any crowd. In no time, Steve was regaling everyone at the table with stories about their high school teachers. He recalled the respect the students had for some teachers and the insolence they showed others. He noted how ironic it was that some of the rowdiest kids ended up as teachers.

Wendy talked about how she had run into a couple of their physical education teachers in the past couple of years. She commented on how "charming" they still were. Charlene said that it was funny how so many of her classmates still couldn't let go of their high school selves.

"What are you, some kind of heathen, Charlene?" Steve said. "You didn't order any meat. You ordered the food that food eats." Charlene did not order an entree with her meal.

"Very funny, Steve," Charlene replied. "I can assure you it's not for religious reasons or because I think getting meat is murder. I do it because I think it's healthier.

"See, for the longest time I blamed my weight on my upbringing," Charlene said. "We were told to clean our plate. We ate sugary cereals for breakfast and fatty foods for dinner. My mom and dad were busy, and it was easier for them to pick up fast food rather than cook. By early grade school I was overweight. I was so uncomfortable and self-conscious in school that I became shy and withdrawn. I hated PE because I felt uncoordinated and dreaded changing clothes in front of people. And I hated school functions, where I was either left out or an afterthought."

"Well, you certainly don't look like that heavy high school girl anymore," Beth said.

"When I was thirty years old I sat around watching television and chowing down on pizza or double cheeseburgers every evening. I was wallowing in my own self-pity. I reluctantly went on a blind date that a co-worker set up for me." She looked at Mike. "We talked about our pastimes, and I said something to the effect that I didn't really have any hobbies. I said that my parents weren't very active in our upbringing, so I never developed any hobbies.

"My sweet future husband looked at me and said, 'You're thirty years old, you haven't been under their legal control for over twelve years. Maybe it's time you stopped blaming your parents, got off your butt, and developed your own hobbies.' Needless to say, the date was not a success.

"I went home, cried, and thought about what that jerk had said. But after a while, I realized he was right. I didn't have to be that maudlin overweight girl anymore. I could be an amiable, happy woman. I joined Toastmasters and a bowling team. I got involved in extracurricular work activities. I was still overweight, but I was happy. I called Mike, my outspoken blind date, and asked him out. We were married a year later.

"About ten years ago, my friend challenged me to a racquetball game. I was still overweight, but I was up to all challenges. I was exhausted after just two points. She had beaten me easily. I decided that I would beat my friend some day. But to do that, I had to get in shape. I went to a spin class four times a week and played racquetball twice a week. My stamina improved, but I couldn't lose weight. She still whipped me.

"So I decided I needed to change how I ate. I loved pepperoni pizzas, cheeseburgers, and beef burritos. I searched and searched for the pepperoni diet to no avail. I found the best way for me to lose weight was to limit the amount of meat I ate. I started losing weight, and pretty soon I was able to beat my friend sometimes. After a couple of years of limiting my meat intake, I just dropped it altogether."

"Without meat, how are you able to get enough protein?" Wendy asked.

"Can someone tell me what you mean by protein?" Beth said what Steve was thinking. "I heard that protein is one of the three macronutrients, along with fat and carbohydrates, but I don't know what protein is or does."

"Proteins[90] are the building blocks of the body," Allan said, jumping in to the conversation. "Protein is constantly being broken down and rebuilt in our bodies.[91] Broken-down proteins are secreted by the liver, the primary organ in charge of protein synthesis, and are either reused or eliminated as waste, primarily in the urine. Because we don't store protein, we need to be continuously ingesting it.[92]

"Have you heard of amino acids?" Allan asked.

They all nodded except for Wendy, who was busy eating, ignoring her husband.

"We have twenty amino acids that link in various ways to make unique proteins with different functions in our body. Eleven amino acids are made inside our body, and therefore we don't need to ingest them. Nine of them are considered essential in that we can get them only through food or supplements.[93]

"The daily recommended amount of protein in a non-pregnant adult is approximately point thirty-seven grams per pound of weight.[94] But this is a rough estimate, and your actual daily needs will depend on your activity level. If you're physically active, you may need as much as point seventy-five grams per pound of body weight."

"I thought I read somewhere that eating too much protein is linked to kidney disease," Charlene said.

"Yes, that's the common perception," Allan said. "While excess protein intake is a concern for persons with pre-existing renal disease, the evidence does not show a link between protein intake and kidney disease in healthy individuals."[95]

"I thought meats like beef, pork, fish, and poultry were where we got our protein," Mike said.

"Animal protein contains the most complete source of protein, which is the most efficiently digested form of protein," Allan explained.

"But herbivores don't have to worry too much, because beans, nuts, and whole grains and even leafy green vegetables like spinach contain protein," Charlene said. "Soy protein and quinoa are considered complete proteins. And you can combine plant foods and ingest your essential amino acids without eating animal products.

"Soy protein is considered a complete protein because it contains most of the essential amino acids found in animal proteins," Charlene continued. "It also contains isoflavones, a chemical compound with beneficial antioxidant effects. There is evidence that soy protein can reduce excess body fat and suppress appetite in obese humans."[96]

"I realize that some protein diets get a bad name," Allan added. "But studies show that high-protein meals suppress later food intake better than low-protein meals of similar caloric intake. Protein shows a stronger effect on a person's desire to eat another meal, called satiety, than meals with higher carbohydrate or fat content. High-protein diets, such as Atkins, Protein Power, and Zone diet have proven to be very effective."[97]

Wendy laughed at the mention of diets. "I love diets. What's the famous quote from Mark Twain about quitting smoking? Oh yeah, 'It's easy to quit smoking. I've done it hundreds of times.' That's how I feel about losing weight. There's not a diet I haven't tried, and they all work. I've lost as few as five pounds and as many as forty-five pounds on half a dozen diets."

"I think it's closer to a dozen diets," Allan said.

Wendy glared at Allan and continued. "Anyway, I lost weight, but as soon as I go off the diet I gain it all back. Sometimes more! Matt told me that you were going to try and lose weight, Steve. Take the advice from a weight-loss pro. Don't bother!" Wendy emphasized her last point by eating a handful of French fries.

"Whoa, there Missy," Allan said, looking embarrassed. Contempt, not hate, is the enemy of most relationships. "Losing weight and keeping it off isn't easy, but don't give up before you even try. If maintaining a healthy weight was easy for you, you would never need to lose weight. Wendy may be right. You may find it easier to lose weight than to keep from regaining it. Some of the factors that play a role in your ability to lose weight and maintain it are your ability to not overeat under regular circumstances. That may mean you need to eat more often, with smaller portions."

Steve thought about his eating habits. He skipped meals and didn't eat until he was famished. He had always finished what was on his plate, because he had been taught it would be rude or inconsiderate to let food go to waste.

"I don't have time to eat a bunch of meals," Steve said. "I get lunch at noon, and then I'm not home until six. If I wake up late, I don't have time for breakfast."

"Keep a protein bar on hand," Allan said, or have almonds or pecans at your desk for those occasions. Drink a large glass of water about thirty minutes before you eat."

There was silence as the group began eating the main entree. Steve's steak looked great. He slathered some butter on his corn and readied fork and knife for the feast.

"I have to admit that in my meat-eating days your meal would have been at the top of my list, Steve," Charlene said. "Unfortunately for you, Steve, there's a week's worth of fat in your meal."

"Susan was telling us to avoid simple carbohydrates," Beth said. "I always thought it was fat that you should avoid."

"I don't think you should avoid fats," Allan said. "Some fats are essential as part of a healthy diet. But at nine calories per gram, fat has more than twice the calories per gram as either protein or carbohydrates. That makes it easy to eat a lot of calories when eating a high-fat meal."

Steve stared at his tasty meal. He pictured a cow laughing at him.

"So are you telling me to eat foods with fat or to avoid them?" Steve asked.

"Both," Allan replied.

"While our body can internally produce most of the fat it needs from non-dietary fat, we need certain essential fatty acids from dietary fats to live," Allan said.[98] "Dietary fats include saturated fats, mono-unsaturated fats, polyunsaturated fats, and trans-fats.

"Most saturated fats are solid at room temperature,"[99] Allan continued. "Foods high in saturated fat include dairy, beef, cocoa butter, and animal and plant fats."

"Saturated fats tend to gravitate toward fat cells," Charlene added, "Therefore, they have been linked to an increased risk of coronary heart disease, including raising total cholesterol and LDL-cholesterol concentrations.[100]

"And while some studies show that certain saturated fat foods do not affect total cholesterol,[101] most studies point toward saturated fats' raising your LDL or bad cholesterol," Charlene said. "If you have to eat foods high in saturated fats like beef and milk products, try to limit it to ten percent or less of your total calories."

"I agree," Allan said. "But I still think you should eat about twenty-five to thirty percent of your calories in fat. You just need to eat the right kind of fat. And if I wanted to cut back on calories, I would be more concerned about simple carbohydrates than I would be about saturated fats of equal caloric value."

"What other types of fat are there?" Beth asked. She had been turning her head from Charlene to Allan as if she were watching a tennis match.

"Monounsaturated fats are liquid at room temperature,"[102] Allan answered. "Olive oil, canola oil, and some fish oils and even avocado are excellent sources of these fats."

"Olive oil is an excellent substitute for butter," Charlene said. "Southern Europeans have been using it for generations. A diet based on monounsaturated fats such as olive oil instead of saturated fats demonstrated a lower risk for cardiovascular disease."[103]

"Yes, olive oil, a famous part of the Mediterranean diet, reduces a number of risk factors for Metabolic Syndrome,"[104] Allan said.

"Canola oil is also an excellent cooking oil," Charlene said. "You would do well if you could replace most of your cooking oils and even the butter you use on bread with olive or canola oils."

"And then there's partially hydrogenated oils,"[105] Allan said.

"What is partially hydrogenated oil?" Beth asked, kicking Steve underneath the table. Steve was distracted by a young boy running among the waiters as they balanced hot trays of food on the palms their hands. His parents were nowhere to be seen. Children are always just seconds away from disaster, he thought.

"What were we talking about?" Steve asked, rubbing his sore shin.

"The infamous transfats,"[106] Charlene said. She was laughing after witnessing the exchange. "Baking products such as shortening and margarine are two types of hydrogenated oils that often contain transfats."

"In a push to increase the shelf life of baked goods, food makers often use transfats," Allan said. "Transfats are found in partially hydrogenated oils and foods made with or fried in them. Because they have been shown to increase cholesterol and triglyceride levels and other markers of cardiovascular disease, I would avoid them. Again, check labels to see if they are included."

"If you're going to start inspecting labels," Charlene said, "you need to be aware of a few things. Food companies are required to list the ingredients on the packages as well as the amount of protein, carbohydrates, and fats. They even list the amount of sugar and types of fats. But they are not required to list the amount of fat if a serving contains less than half a gram of it. The trick is to have a serving size small enough so that the amount of fat, or in this case transfat, is less than half a gram. If it is, they can make the claim that it doesn't contain transfats."

"The same goes for sugar," Allan said. "Sugar-free simply means that a serving contains less than half a gram of sugar."

"On the one hand, you tell me that transfats are bad for us," Steve said, "and on the other, you're telling us that we could be eating them without know it?"

Charlene nodded. "First, look at the ingredients. If it contains hydrogenated or partially hydrogenated vegetable oil, it probably has transfats. Most margarines and shortenings have transfats. And lots of commercially baked cookies and crackers contain transfats. Another form of hidden fat that you can find on labels is monoglycerides and diglycerides. These are forms of fat that are not counted as calories on the label but contain calories nonetheless."

"While we're on the subject of labels," Allan said, "pay attention to serving sizes. The food item may appear to be light in calories, but the serving size is so small a hummingbird couldn't live off of it. You buy a twenty-ounce drink. You look on the label, and it states that a serving contains eighty calories. Look closer, and a serving is only eight ounces. That means that it is two hundred calories in total."

Steve's head was spinning. Limit saturated fat to ten percent of my daily calories, he thought, and avoid transfats and foods with partially dehydrogenated oils. And read labels.

He excused himself to use the restroom. He started to head toward the corral, but decided to fight his instincts to treat the event like a camping trip. The restrooms were in the back of the restaurant, so he passed dining patrons. He dodged the five-year-old and a couple of other children using the restaurant as their personal playground.

Normally he wouldn't pay attention to the diners, but with all of the talk about food he eyed the people devouring their meal. They looked like lions feasting on a wildebeest after a three-day fast. He thought about how he treated a night out at a nice restaurant. He would purposely not eat all day in order to have room for more food. He wondered if the diners even tasted their food.

He shuddered when he returned to his table, because he noticed that he had cleaned his plate.

"Don't go back there," Steve said. "One of those guys was eyeing my arm as he was opening a bottle of steak sauce."

Did you say that some fat is good for you?" Steve asked, feeling a little excited after his excursion.

"Yes," Allan replied. "There are two types of fat that are considered essential because we must get them through our diet. They are Omega-six fats and Omega-three fats.

"Omega-six fats are found in poultry, pork, and beef and in sunflower, safflower, corn, cotton seed, and soybean oils. Among other things, they play an important role in the health of our cell membranes.[107]

"The other essential fats are Omega-three fatty acids, which are found in fish, flaxseeds, and walnuts.[108] They form a part of cell membranes in the brain and eyes. They regulate blood clotting and play an anti-inflammatory role in our body. They decrease Metabolic Syndrome factors by stimulating fat oxidation, reducing body fat, and raising anti-inflammatory markers.[109] Fish is our best dietary source of omega-three fats. Also, fish consumption has been shown to reduce the risk of strokes."[110]

"As a vegetarian, I take flaxseed oil for Omega-three supplementation," Charlene said. "Flaxseed oil contains alphalinolenic acid, or ALA. It's another form of Omega-three fatty acid."

"From my research, the Omega-three fatty acid found in flaxseed oil responds differently from the Omega-three fatty acid found in fish,"[111] Allan said.

"Flaxseed oil is not as efficient as fish oil, so I just take a higher amount of it," Charlene replied.

Allan nodded and continued. "Regardless of how you get your omega-three fatty acid, it is extremely important to get sufficient amounts of it, because even the ratio of omega-three fats to omega-six fats appears to be important."

"What do you mean by the ratio?" Steve asked.

"I mean that you would benefit from ingesting more omega-three fat because that will reduce your risk of cardiovascular disease, coronary heart disease, and depression."[112,113]

"It sounds like the fatty acid that I need to be concerned with are the Omega-three ones. Steve said.

"They're both important, but unless you're a fish eater, like me," Allan said, eating his salmon, "you will need to consider supplementing your diet with Omega-three fatty acids. I recommend taking at least fifteen hundred milligrams. If you eat a large amount of foods that contain Omega-six fatty acids such as corn or soy, you may want to consider increasing the amount of Omega-three fatty acids to over two thousand milligrams."

"I take about eight thousand milligrams of flaxseed oil a day," Charlene said.

Steve leaned back in his chair. He felt his meal settling in his stomach.

"If we're going to talk about fat, we might as well talk about cholesterol," Charlene said.

"Our body produces all of the cholesterol we need, so it's not an essential part of our diet," Allan explained. "Meat, poultry, fish, and dairy products contain dietary cholesterol. Plant foods do not contain cholesterol. Most of the foods that contain it also contain saturated fat, so it's difficult to measure the effects of dietary cholesterol on blood levels of cholesterol, and other markers for cardiovascular disease are mixed.

"Dietary cholesterol does not appear to be as harmful as transfats or saturated fat since it seems to raise blood cholesterol in only one of three people and only if ingested above three hundred milligrams, or about two eggs," Allan said.

Steve was still thinking about steak. "I thought steak was mostly protein," he said. "Why all the talk about fat?"

"Yes, protein is the primary nutrient in your steak, Steve," Allan agreed. "But your steak also contains a significant amount of saturated fat. Since we're on the subject, let's look at your meal."

Steve sighed and stared at his empty plate.

"You had a salad as a starter," Allan said. "With cucumbers, tomatoes, and lettuce, it had the potential of being healthy. But each tablespoon of ranch dressing contains over seventy calories. Almost ninety percent of ranch dressing's calories come from fat, and there is even some transfat in it. I would guess that you had at least two tablespoons of it in your salad. A vinegar and oil dressing is a much healthier alternative."

"You ordered two side dishes: garlic mashed potatoes and corn on the cob. A baked potato would have been a better choice. A baked potato has more fiber as well as potassium and vitamins C and B$_6$. Garlic mashed potatoes removes the skin, which contains a lot of the nutrients, and adds milk or half and half and thus increases the saturated fat content. Sweet potatoes would be much better for you.

"Corn is a vegetable that is a decent source of vitamins and minerals. An ear of corn is about seventy-five calories, but you can double that with saturated fat if you add butter to it. The green beans are a better choice, because they're high in nutrients and fiber, but corn is much better than French fries. No offense, Wendy."

Wendy had stopped paying attention to the conversation. She was watching a group attempting to line dance. Alcohol masked a dearth of rhythm and coordination, she thought.

"I won't tell you to never eat steak," Allan continued, "but I would limit the amount to about four ounces and not add butter or a similar substance to it. If you have a choice, go with lean cuts of turkey or chicken or best of all fish such as salmon. But the biggest calorie addition you made was adding béarnaise sauce to your steak. It consisted of almost pure saturated fat.

"Your choice of ranch dressing in the salad, milk in the potatoes, butter on the corn, and béarnaise sauce on the steak increased the number of calories by about fifty percent while adding very little nutritional value."

"I'm sorry to be the bearer of bad news, Steve," Allan said.

Until this weekend, Steve hadn't thought about what he ate except to eat what tasted good. He didn't think of food as healthy or unhealthy.

"That's okay, Allan," he said. "I'm not a finicky eater. I just have to make some easy substitutions and change from eating poorly to eating lower-calorie, nutritious meals."

Allan agreed.

After dinner, Beth and Steve were free to mingle. They reluctantly joined the line-dancing crew. Despite their initial trepidation, they had a great time tripping over their own feet and bumping into their friends.

They ended the evening talking to some couples about children. Two of his classmates had children in college. Steve talked about becoming an empty nester. His youngest was ten, but as Beth attested, time flies, and before they knew it the house would be empty and quiet.

As they walked back to their room, Beth brought up the subject discussed during dinner.

"That was a nice meal," she said. "Although I was kind of expecting Wendy to plunge her steak knife into Allan."

Steve chuckled. "I think she would have except that it would have ruined her dinner."

"Anyway, I learned a lot tonight," Steve said. "I didn't know that active people could eat up to point seventy-five grams of protein per pound or that poultry and even beans and vegetables were excellent sources of essential amino acids."

"Who would have guessed that not all fats are bad," Beth said. "I like fish, and if I didn't, I think I would get an Omega-three supplement."

"I'm bummed about steak," Steve said, "but at least I can eat it in limited amounts as long as I eat ten percent or fewer of my calories in saturated fat like butter."

"Speaking of fats, I'm going to look at our food labels and see if we have any transfats either labeled or hidden," Beth said. "And I will see how many calories there are per serving."

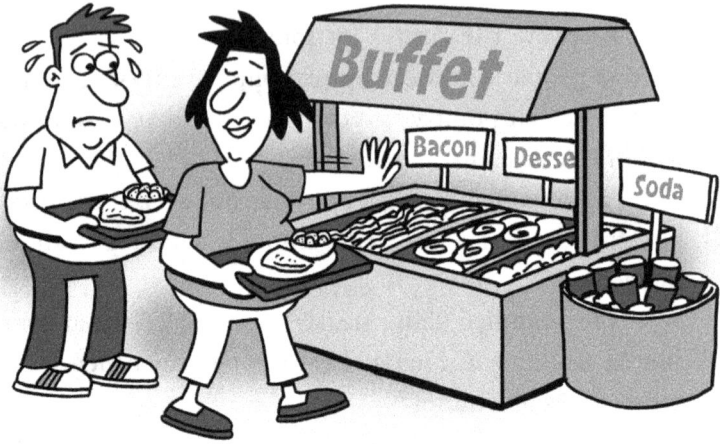

# 11

## VITAMINS AND MINERALS

Beth's and Steve's flight didn't leave until noon, so they had time to enjoy the Sunday morning brunch at one of the resort's restaurants. Brunch was a buffet complete with an omelet station and a vast assortment of fruits, precooked meats, and breads. Buffets were big-eater's delights. But even light eaters were hard-pressed not to overindulge, because it was tempting to "get your money's worth."

Steve eyed the array of foods. His breakfast usually consisted of a soft drink and a candy bar, bagel, or muffin. Of course he didn't usually have a team of cooks to make his meals. He planned on making a change in his breakfast after speaking with Beth about what Laurie had told her. But now a buffet stared at him, and he knew that he wouldn't eat again until he got back home after a three-hour flight. With the drive time and the wait at the airport, it would be at least six hours before he ate anything but peanuts or pretzels.

He decided to indulge because he wasn't planning to change his eating habits until at least Monday. Besides, the buffet was not cheap. He ordered a cheese-and-bacon omelet, sausage, and sourdough toast.

He eyed the pancakes but decided to skip them for now. Beth and Steve were searching for a seat when Marcia waved them down.

Marcia had a small plate with a single egg white and some fruit and vegetables. Steve thought about the money she was wasting at the buffet.

Based on the large pile of food on Ivan's plate, it was clear that he had decided on the buffet.

"Shouldn't you be getting more food at the price of the buffet? Steve asked.

"I ordered from the menu," Marcia said. "You didn't have to get the buffet, Steve."

"We don't get to dine at resort restaurants very often," Beth said. "We decided that Steve was going to start his diet next week."

"This may seem trivial, Beth," Marcia said, "but I would focus on a change of eating habits rather than putting Steve on a diet."

After they sat down, Marcia swallowed some pills.

"What's with the pills?" Steve asked.

"The bariatric surgery Ivan and I had shrunk our stomachs and decreased the time our bodies had to digest food. This made it difficult to absorb all of the vitamins and minerals we need," Marcia explained. "Therefore, we were required to take supplements. I take some extra ones because I think they're helpful."

"Should we be taking vitamin and mineral supplements?" Steve asked.

"Vitamins and minerals are micronutrients that support essential functions in the body,"[114] Marcia said. "You can get an adequate amount of most vitamins and minerals by eating correctly. They're absorbed in your body more efficiently if you ingest them with food. Fruits and vegetables are great sources. But even if I didn't have to take supplements, I would still take certain vitamins and minerals despite the fact that I eat a well-balanced diet."

"What would the different vitamins do for me?"

"Vitamins A, C, and E are antioxidants that will help clean out free radicals and reduce inflammation. They have upper limits, but even with a healthy diet of fruits and vegetables, vitamin supplements won't be harmful.

"Regardless of whether you take a multiple vitamin, I would take a vitamin D supplement. Vitamin D, like vitamins A, E, and K, is a fat-soluble vitamin. It's required for normal calcium and phosphorus metabolism. As such it is important for musculoskeletal health. A vitamin D deficiency has been linked to insulin resistance, obesity — primarily visceral fat—and other metabolic syndrome symptoms."[115],[116]

"What foods do I need to eat so that I don't have a deficiency?" Beth asked.

"The primary source of vitamin D is exposure to the ultraviolet radiation of the sun," Marcia replied. "It's taken from the skin and stored in fat. Absorption through the skin is affected by atmospheric conditions, clothing, sunscreen, the amount of melanin in the skin, body mass, and age. People with darker skin and those who live in colder climates tend to have a greater percentage of vitamin D deficiency."[117]

"How much vitamin D should I take?" Beth asked.

"The recommended daily amount is six hundred IUs a day for adults under the age of seventy-one and eight hundred IUs for adults over the age of seventy-one. I take about two thousand IUs a day."

"I have a friend who got a vitamin B shot the other day," Steve said.

"I've heard of vitamin $B_{12}$ shots," Marcia said. "The B vitamins are not fat-soluble. If you fail to eat foods that contain those nutrients for a couple of days, you may become deficient in them. Again, although I eat a healthy diet, I take B-complex vitamins. B vitamins aid in metabolism of fats, proteins, and carbohydrates, and they aid in red cell production and help your immune system and your nervous system.

"Vitamin $B_{12}$—cobalamins—is a water-soluble vitamin that helps metabolize folic acid to build DNA, aids in neurological function, and helps in the formation of blood cells.[118] Foods that contain $B_{12}$ include poultry, fish, shellfish, and dairy products. Because it's found mostly in animal foods, vegetarians need to be careful to either eat sufficient amounts of vitamin $B_{12}$ or takes supplements. Maybe your friend was a vegetarian, or perhaps his doctor felt that he needed the boost in metabolism and energy.

"You can also have deficiencies in other B vitamins," Marcia continued. "Deficiencies in thiamin, or Vitamin $B_1$, may cause fatigue, memory impairment, and irritability. Vitamin $B_1$ is found in beans, meats, cereal grains, and nuts.

"Vitamin $B_3$—niacin—is a water-soluble vitamin that, like the other B vitamins, is instrumental in metabolism.[119] Foods that contain niacin include poultry, fish, cereal, eggs, and nuts.

"Folic acid, or folate, is another water-soluble vitamin that helps metabolize proteins, form red blood cells, synthesize and repair DNA, and promote cell growth and division.[120] Foods that contain folic acid include citrus fruits, legumes, leafy vegetables, and sunflower seeds. It is also often added to white flour.

"Choline is a water-soluble nutrient that is still waiting official induction into the B-vitamin class. It aids in the transportation of very low-density lipoproteins through our blood system, thus lowering cholesterol.[121] Foods containing choline include eggs, liver, and chicken. Vegetarians may find it difficult to ingest sufficient amounts of choline without supplementation."

Steve had finished his first course and was eyeing the waffles. Beth took notes as she ate. It would take Steve some time to absorb the information, but right now he was contemplating getting his money's worth at the expensive buffet.

"I understand you paid a lot for the buffet, so it seems like a waste of money not to take advantage of the all-you-can-eat aspect of it," Marcia said, reading Steve's mind. "Ivan and I would revolve our schedule around inexpensive all-you-can-eat -style restaurants. But I can't emphasize enough the need to downsize your meals. It will be difficult at first since you're used to a starve-and-binge lifestyle. Just remember, most restaurants are all-you-can-eat. They give you such large portions that you're overfull if you finish it. Unfortunately, we're also trained to clean our plate. If you don't figure out a way to either avoid places like that or eat half or less than half of the meal and take the rest home, you are destined to remain heavy."

Shoot! Steve thought. He didn't know if he was really hungry, but he also loved waffles and maple syrup.

"How about this, Steve," Marcia said, placing her hand on his arm. "Wait five minutes. If you're hungry, then go get the waffles or pancakes you're eyeballing."

Steve reluctantly agreed.

"What about minerals?" Beth asked. "Do I need to take a mineral supplement, too?"

"Most multivitamins contain minerals," Marcia replied. "There are a number of essential minerals that our body does not produce in adequate quantities without getting them from the food we eat. Minerals include calcium, magnesium, sodium, sulfur, potassium, chromium, phosphorus, and chloride, plus the trace minerals copper, zinc, fluoride, cobalt, manganese, molybdenum, iodine, and selenium."

"That's a bunch!" Steve said.

"I agree, and that's only a partial list," Marcia said. "However, most minerals are found in adequate supply in even the most rudimentary diet and, therefore, you don't need to think about them when considering the foods you're eating or supplementation."

"Which ones do I need to supplement, or do I need to worry about it if I just get a multi-vitamin?" Steve asked.

"The four I think you need to consider supplementing are calcium, magnesium, iron, and zinc

"Calcium is the primary nutrient found in our bones and teeth. It is also essential for blood vessel dilation and contraction, muscle contraction, and nerve transmission. Calcium deficiencies can lead to bone loss and osteoporosis. Dairy products, tofu, salmon, yogurt, soy milk, and spinach are a few foods rich in calcium. If you eat dairy, then you shouldn't need a supplement.

"Magnesium is needed to make several enzymes. It aids in maintaining nerve function and in energy production. It is also thought to play a role in regulating blood pressure and sugar levels.

Cashews, almonds, halibut, spinach, and nuts are a few of the foods rich in magnesium.

"Iron is essential to the transport of oxygen in our blood system. Inadequate amounts of iron can lead to fatigue and anemia. Pregnant women should consult their doctor regarding iron supplementation. Iron is found in meat sources, called heme irons, or plant sources, called non-heme irons. It is easier to absorb heme irons than non-heme irons. Heme irons are found in poultry, beef, shellfish, and fish. Non-heme irons are found in oatmeal, soy beans, lentils, and some fortified cereals.

"Zinc is an essential trace element that plays a role in our immune system. It is needed in the breakdown and buildup of a number of enzymes. Zinc is also needed for protein metabolism and cell growth and division. But don't take too much zinc. Large amounts of zinc, even as much as a hundred fifty milligrams can cause nausea, abdominal cramps, and vomiting and can lead to a copper deficiency.[122]

"Zinc is found in abundance in oysters and in decent amounts in other animal products. It is found in limited amounts in plant foods and, therefore, vegetarians may have difficulty ingesting an adequate amount without supplementation."

"It seems like I can get all of the vitamins and minerals I need from food," Beth said.

"You're able to eat and drink all of the nutrients you need for a healthy lifestyle," Marcia said. "The only vitamin that is difficult to get in food is vitamin D. The only macronutrients that may be difficult to get in diet are Omega-three fatty acids. Vegetarians may have a difficult time getting enough Vitamin $B_{12}$, choline, hemi-iron, and zinc. But some research suggests that multivitamin and mineral supplements may have a positive effect on mood, stress, and cognitive function in middle-age males.[123]

"I have to take a supplement because of my surgery. Had I not had the surgery, I would still take a daily vitamin as well as a B-complex vitamin, a D vitamin, an Omega-three fatty acid and CoQ-ten supplements."

"I listen to talk radio," Steve said. "On Sunday mornings the airwaves are full of shows selling the latest supplement that will help me lose weight, swim across the channel from England to France, and have the energy and libido to sleep with all the women when I reach the other side."

"Sign me up," said Ivan, jumping into the conversation. He was torturing Steve with his pastry dessert.

"We're just beginning to understand how the body processes the millions of chemicals in our body," Marcia said as she wearily stares at Ivan shoveling in the last morsel of food. "There are a number of nutrients that may provide great benefits to our bodies, including the digestive, cardiovascular, and respiratory systems. But be wary of cure-alls. Radio, television, and the Internet are rife with quick fixes that make grand claims. Many are the twenty-first century's equivalent of the nineteenth century's snake oil salesman selling elixirs aimed to remedy your every ill. The Internet is a great tool for research, but it is rampant with misinformation."

Marcia had pushed her plate away with part of her egg uneaten. After waiting, Steve found that he was full and was glad he didn't eat more food. But he's still thinking about the delicious pastry Ivan had demolished.

They finished their meal and said their good-byes.

As Steve and Beth walked back to their room, they passed the hotel gym. Some type of class had just ended, and they saw Mike, Charlene's husband, walk out sweating. Mike was a big guy and not the type Steve would picture doing aerobics, so he stopped to talk to him.

"Hey, Mike," Steve said. "Were you taking some sort of boxing aerobics class?"

"No, I was taking a yoga class."

"Yoga, seriously?"

"Yes, yoga," Mike said, looking annoyed. "I dare you to try it for fifteen minutes. I used to play basketball, but it was too hard on my knees. A friend suggested I try yoga. I had the same response as yours.    I did my own research and found that yoga is a great combination of physical endurance, strength, and flexibility."

"I've talked to a couple of people about strength and endurance training, but I haven't heard anyone mention flexibility training," Steve said.

"Flexibility training will improve posture, increase your range of motion, increase the blood flow to your muscles, and reduce your risk of injury," Mike said.   "You can perform routine stretching exercises that you can find on the Internet. You could also do Pilates. I like yoga because it offers an excellent variety of flexibility, strength, and endurance training.  Also, yoga has excellent breathing techniques that help you to relax."

"Hmm, I always saw yoga as something women did," Steve said.

Mike smiled. "Exactly."

As they walked away, Beth said to Steve, "Supplements and stretching.  One day you will be the modern-day Jack LaLane."

Steve laughed.   "I would be fine being the thirty-year-old Steve."

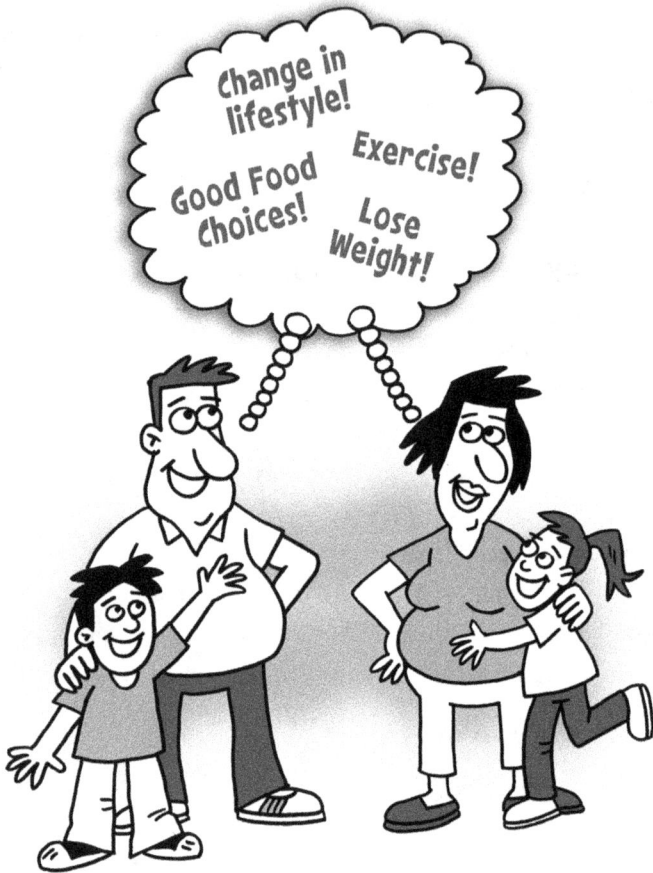

# 12

## THE FLIGHT HOME

Steve and Beth took a taxi to the airport. They made it through the TSA gauntlet, boarded the plane, and headed back to Seattle. Steve thought about his test results and the information he had heard that weekend. It seemed clear that he needed to change his eating habits and start to exercise.

A familiar voice interrupted his thoughts.

"Hi, guys." It was Paul, the same person they had flown with to Phoenix. "How was the reunion?"

"We're getting old," Steve said with a laugh.

"Every day above ground is a good day," Paul replied.

"Would you mind sitting with us?" Beth said. "We heard a lot of information about food and exercise, so we'd love to talk to you about it."

Paul agreed, wondering if they were just trying to get away from the guy in their row who smelled as if he was allergic to water.

"Well," Paul said as he sat down, "did you discover the magic pill that will allow you to live life as usual and rid yourself of that dastardly Metabolic Syndrome?"

"No, I had no such luck," Steve said. "But I did learn that I eat like crap and I need to start exercising."

"How do you eat like crap?" Paul asked.

"To start with, my breakfast sets me up to be tired and hungry by late morning." Laurie, a friend of ours, told Beth that she thinks breakfast is the most important meal of the day. She advised eating fruits and maybe an egg white. She said that the simple sugars I have in a soft drink and donut or candy bar give me quick energy that won't last, increase the likelihood of becoming insulin-resistant, and add to potential weight gain."

"Does that about sum it up, Beth?" Steve said, turning to Beth.

"That's about right," Beth replied. "She said that it should be the biggest meal of the day but low in fat and sugar."

"Actually, I wouldn't advise describing a meal as bigger than the next one," Paul said. "It should range from three hundred to four hundred calories and should be low in saturated fat and simple carbohydrates."

"That's right," Steve said excitedly. "No meals bigger than a fist. That tidbit came from Marcia, a friend who had gastric bypass surgery."

"And our doctor friend, Susan, said I should have some type of midmorning snack. She suggested almonds or walnuts, I think."

"Fruit or a protein bar make excellent snacks, too," Paul said. "Almonds and walnuts are great, but don't eat too many because they're dense. Limit the almonds, pecans, or walnuts to half a cup."

"I'm going to try and go without wheat, because I think that I may be gluten-intolerant," Beth said.

"What makes you think that?"

"I told Laurie about how I was tired and irritable all the time."

"How old are you?" Paul asked. Paul's bedside manner called for a direct approach without suffering inconsequential niceties.

Beth was slightly startled at the direct question, but she said "I'm forty-eight."

"I don't think it would hurt to go gluten-free," Paul said. "Steve, you could do the same thing and see if you feel better. The fact is we don't always know the long-term effects foods have on us until we eliminate them. But I would also get your blood checked to see if you have any hormonal imbalances. People your age or even younger commonly have a hormonal imbalance. Go to a specialist and have him check your testosterone, estrogen, progesterone, DHEA, and thyroid levels. "

"Susan also advised us not to drink our calories," Steve said. "Does that mean I should switch to diet drinks?"

"I would drink water or green tea," Paul replied. "Some studies suggest that drinking artificially sweetened drinks may lead to eating more calories. And we don't know if there is a link between artificial sweeteners and some forms of cancer. But if you must drink soft drinks, I would drink diet sodas instead of regular ones."

"Speaking of soft drinks," Steve said, "I was advised to limit my sugar intake."

"The recommended daily allowance for sugar is forty grams," Paul said. "If you start counting calories—something I would advocate at least initially—you will be shocked at how much sugar you consume.

"In fact," Paul continued, "I would speculate that if most people who were overweight simply limited their intake of sugars and simple carbohydrates, they would lose weight, lower their blood glucose levels and other Metabolic Syndrome factors, and feel better."

"What about excessive saturated fat?" Beth asked. "Yeah, I was told to limit my saturated fat intake to ten percent of my daily intake," Steve said.

"Sure, saturated fat may be bad because foods high in saturated fat tend to be calorie-dense, and they have been linked to cardiovascular disease and a rise in LDL cholesterol. But don't substitute high-fat foods for high-sugar foods. The best way to limit your saturated fat intake is to read labels and avoid creamy foods. Most extra calories in foods are not the primary food but what is added to it. Oils are added to make fried foods, creamy dressings are added to salad to ruin an otherwise nutritious meal, and sour cream and butter are added to potatoes. Lard or other high-fat oils are added to beans. If you use oils to cook, substitute corn oil or peanut oil with canola oil or extra-virgin olive oil.

"Did you talk to anyone about exercise?" Paul asked.

"Yes, we talked about three ways of losing or maintaining my weight," Steve replied.

"Three?"

"Yes," Steve said, pleased he might know something this doctor didn't know. "A thing called NEAT, resistance exercise, and aerobic exercise."

"What is NEAT?"

"I can't remember what the acronym stands for, but it's the calories we use when we aren't sitting, digesting food, or exercising on purpose. I believe that NEAT includes gardening or other yard work, physical work done on the job, housework, walking the dog, walking to and from the car, and even standing."

Paul laughed. "I guess you call that the fidgeters revenge."

Steve smiled at that. "I talked to Rob about resistance training."

Paul didn't say anything. It didn't look as if Steve had done a lot of resistance training.

"He suggested I do some form of resistance training at least twice a week on non-consecutive days," Steve said. "I used to be into weightlifting, but I may look at machine weights or even body-resistance programs."

"My friends Rob and Matt took me on a hike and discussed aerobic exercise. I'm definitely out of shape. We went for a short hike, and I almost didn't make it. They suggested I find an aerobic activity to do at least four days a week for a minimum of half an hour at a time."

"I think you should try for six days a week for forty minutes to an hour," Paul said.

"We also ran into a classmate's husband right after a yoga class. He said that it's a great combination of resistance, aerobics, and flexibility training."

"Yoga may be a good idea, as it may relieve stress, too," Paul said. "Stress also affects our response to foods. Stress makes about two-thirds of us eat more, and everyone else eat less.[124] Even those who don't overeat tend to eat pleasure foods that are high in fat or sugar. For reasons still unknown, pleasure foods appear to reduce the feeling of being stressed."[125]

Paul didn't say anything for a while. He wasn't a weight-loss professional, but because of his specialty he dealt a lot with patients who needed to lose weight.

"Sounds like you had a very informative weekend," Paul said. "I thought you'd probably blown it off this weekend because you were on vacation. It says a lot that you took the opportunity to learn something about exercise and food.

"I realize you haven't asked, but I'm going to offer my advice anyway. As you can see from my physique, I don't do a lot of resistance training, so take this for whatever it's worth. Initially, I focused on aerobic training. I think you need to get your weight down to a manageable amount before worrying about increasing muscle mass. You need to properly warm up and cool down, which includes stretching. Concentrate on working toward exercising an hour a day, six days a week. You may find that you're tired after twenty minutes. It's okay to slow down and even to rest.

"Once you have your weight down to below two hundred pounds, which may take a few months, then look into adding resistance training. When you do more research, you will find a lot of support for high-intensity, short-duration training. I have no doubt that you can burn a lot of calories that way. But I question the ability to maintain the intensity long-term.

"And if you aren't looking at this as a life change, you're all but wasting your time. That's why you need to find an activity you enjoy. Or find a variety of activities you enjoy. Try aerobics, swimming, boxing, running, or biking. If you don't enjoy it, you won't continue it.

"Either find a reliable partner or, if you're going to exercise on your own, make an appointment with yourself. It should be as important as family and as work. You won't do either one of them any good if you're dead or incapacitated."

That last sentence dropped onto Steve and Beth like an anvil. Steve had almost forgotten why he had gone on his information quest in the first place.

"Based on my medical records, it doesn't look like I have much choice but to become healthier," Steve said.

"You do have a choice. Many people facing your situation or worse choose to do nothing," Paul said. "If you have decided to make a change, you have to decide how you're going to go about it. You need to assess your own personality to decide if you're a self-starter who is able to lose weight and maintain the weight or if you need help. Almost every successful weight loser used a combination of diet and exercise to keep the weight off. Three out of four weighed themselves at least once a week. Breakfast was a main meal in about four out of five of the successful weight losers. Finally, consistent eating habits were a major factor in their success."[126]

"Do you think I should do one of those diets where I buy their food?" Steve asked.

"It isn't a bad way to jump-start your weight loss. The reputable ones provide an assortment of foods, and they tend to be nutritious. They have proven to be more successful than if you used your own plan at losing weight and keeping it off.[127] If you follow the plan, you will lose weight."

"What if he decides to lose weight on his own?" Beth asked.

"There are two ways to 'go it alone,'" Paul replied. "You can eat fewer calories but maintain a healthy diet, or you can do some form of starvation diet or a diet that misses key nutrients. If your diet consists of eating well-rounded, healthy meals and exercising, I think it's a great way to lose weight. You will develop healthy habits that will provide a template for a new lifestyle. But unmonitored diets that limit or even eliminate key nutrients can be counterproductive and even dangerous.

"Based on what you told me about your trip, you have what it takes to go it alone. But regardless of which route you decide to take, make a commitment to yourself but involve others. View it as a lifestyle change and not just a temporary fix. If you don't, you will be just like most overweight and obese people who gain back about one-third of their lost weight within one year and gain all of it back within three to five years.[128]

"Beth, you can be a help or a hindrance to Steve's success. Social support will play a role in Steve's ability to lose weight and to maintain the weight loss. Weight-loss clinics provide support, but the more important support will need to come from family and friends."

"Social support," Steve said with a laugh. "I go out with my buddies and order a spritzer, and I'll get laughed out of the room."

"If you can't take some guff from your friends, you have issues that go beyond weight," Paul said. "First, I would solicit your friends in your effort. They can be a benefit instead of a hindrance. Second, if they're genuinely offended by changes you need to make in order to give you a longer, healthier life, you may want to reconsider your definition of a friend. And third, you may find it easier to avoid the places or situations where you are likely to overindulge for a while. But if you're going to be successful at making a change, you will need to learn to embrace those situations in a positive way. Try to mentally prepare for the situations with a positive response."

"What can I do to help?" Beth asked.

"You can be a positive influence. That doesn't mean you need to follow his eating or exercising plans, but if you did, it would make it easier for him. It does mean helping him with food choices. You both can go through your pantry, freezer, and refrigerator and pick out healthy foods and foods he will want to limit or eliminate. I would mark them as healthy— Eat anytime, Decent—eat a small portion, and

Unhealthy— don't eat or eat rarely. Also, choose restaurants where the healthy choices are easy and accessible.

"If Steve chooses to enter an open-water swimming event, work with him on his training schedule. When Steve eats or drinks foods that are not on his preferred list, he needs to treat it like a bump in the road and not a roadblock. The greatest chance of success will be if he embraces his lifestyle and doesn't view it as punishment.

"If you, Steve, view this as punishment for years of abuse, you will do your penance and then go back to your old ways. Experiment with different healthy-eating alternatives and exercises until you find ones you enjoy. If you find them, your chances of success are much better.

"Finally, don't jump into a diet tonight. Plan and prepare for it. Set a date like next Saturday or Sunday to start. Talk to each other, your children, and your friends about it. Prepare your kitchen and pantry with foods and decide on your exercise regimen. Your chances of success increase if you place yourself in a position where you're adequately prepared to act."

Paul decided it was time to jump off his soap box. He enjoyed talking to people about health when he felt they were genuinely interested in it. He thought Beth and Steve were at that point. Of course everyone's a hero until the first shot is fired. He had seen many short-term triumphs that became long-term failures. He didn't know if Steve would successfully lose the weight and keep it off, but he hoped he would.

They said their good-byes at the baggage claim carousel. They exchanged business cards, and Paul asked Steve to keep him abreast of his progress.

Steve and Beth didn't say anything on the way home. Beth was excited about the lifestyle change, but she didn't want to be too enthusiastic, because Steve might think she was unhappy with the way he was now. She also planned to get her blood tested and to read more about gluten intolerance food allergies.

Steve thought about the changes he needed to make. He had decided to go on his own initially, but he wanted to make sure he proceeded in a way that would increase his chances of success. He found a cell phone app that would help him count calories, and he thought he was disciplined enough to change his eating and exercise habits without help.

Beth thought about the foods they had at home. She would go through the kitchen and pantry and see which foods were healthy and which ones were empty calorie bombs.

When they arrived at their house, they heard the dog barking, but otherwise the house was quiet. They opened the door to a dog who acted as if she had just found her long-lost best friend who'd been missing for years. Sara yelled "Daddy!" and jumped into Steve's arms. Zack nodded at them as he texted. How quickly children change, Steve thought. Time marches on, and they'll be gone before you can blink.

Steve said his hellos, entered the kitchen, and opened the refrigerator. He hadn't eaten since brunch. He inspected the choices staring back at him. It was the same array of foods that had stared at him when he left.

He gave himself a week to put together a workable diet and exercise plan.

# Epilogue

## Steve's Plan

Steve did not immediately start a new eating and exercise regimen. Jumping into a major life change without adequate preparation invites failure. He spent the first week preparing himself and his family and friends. He decided to make a list of high-nutrition foods such as lean proteins, whole grains, vegetables and real fruit and take note of the ones he liked. He also made a list of foods to avoid such as refined carbohydrates and foods high in saturated fats. Beth agreed to follow the eating plan as support for Steve. They didn't want to make any major changes to Zack's and Sara's eating habits, so some of the foods on Steve's avoid list would remain in the house but he would mark them with a red pen as a reminder to not eat them.

Steve decided to discuss his plan with his friends and co-workers. He made a commitment to them and asked that they support him. He advised his friends and family that it might take him some time to adjust, so they had to be patient with him. Their support was important to his success.

Steve decided to record his weight, waist measurement, and waist to hip ratio. He also began tracking his eating habits. He tried to keep track of how much he ate, when he ate and how he felt before and after eating.

## The first couple of weeks

Initially, the food and exercise would be difficult. He was changing years of habits. His body would react. He might feel queasy. Some of the foods would be foreign to his taste buds as well as his stomach. He would start an exercise program. His muscles would be angry. His lungs might go on strike.

After a week of making the food changes, it should become easier. His body would begin adjusting to the new nutrients, and he would begin to develop a routine. But it's important that Steve doesn't get frustrated if it remains difficult. He might need to try different foods or combinations of foods that are on the list.

## What to eat

Steve would eat whole fresh foods and avoid or limit processed and refined foods. He would do this by spending a majority of his grocery shopping time in the produce section. He had decided to eat a nutritious breakfast. Instead of eating two or three large meals a day, he would eat small meals five times a day. Eating every few hours would keep him from feeling famished and rushing to the ice cream parlor. He would not eat shortly before going to sleep, because food digestion inhibits sleep. He would drink a glass of water about twenty minutes before eating to decrease his hunger.

Water is critical. While most of the foods we eat contain water, it is not enough to keep us hydrated. Dehydration can make you lethargic. It makes it more difficult to digest your food. It will make exercise and even your daily activities more difficult.[129] As little as a 2% decrease in hydration can lead to reduced cognitive function.[130] The exact amount of water you need varies depending on your activity level and what else you are drinking. However, a safe amount of water is about 0.6 ounces for every pound you weigh.

Steve decided to track his food and drinks so that would have a better idea of the amount of calories he was ingesting. Since his predicted daily caloric expenditure is approximately 2,500 calories a day, he would initially eat approximately 1,750 calories a day. This would lead to loss of about one and a half pounds a week. Once he reached his optimal weight he would increase his caloric intake but keep eating the same healthier foods.

He would track his progress by weighing himself once a week at the same time of day.

## Example of daily eating plan and supplements
**Breakfast:** 2 boiled eggs, a piece of whole grain toast with olive oil, an orange and green tea (350 calories)
**Snack:** Two servings of almonds or walnuts and an apple (280 calories)
**Lunch:** Romaine lettuce salad with chicken, tomatoes, and peas with oil-and-vinegar dressing (350 calories)
**Snack:** A protein bar and grapes (280 calories)
**Dinner:** Grilled salmon and asparagus with whole-grain rice and black beans (385 calories)

## Exercise
Steve would either bike or take a spin class five days a week for at least forty minutes. On weekends he could substitute his biking for hiking with his family. He would do a resistance-training regimen consisting of pushups, pull-ups, lunges, and wall squats twice a week for at least half an hour each time. He decided to exercise in the morning before work since he was busy with family events after work.

He also decided to do his own lawn work with help from Beth, Zack, and Sara. In addition to spending quality time with his family, this would significantly increase his calorie burn rate compared to his traditional routine of drinking beer and watching sports. He would choose parking spaces that required more walking; he would stand or pace when he was on the phone; and he would stand while working at his desk for part of his day. He purchased a pedometer so that he could track the number of steps he took in a day.

## Success tips
Steve would plan his meals ahead of time so that he didn't cupboard-hunt when he felt hungry. He went online and searched for nutritious alternatives at the restaurants he went to with his co-workers at lunch and friends at dinner. If he wasn't familiar with the

restaurant, he would ask the server for healthy substitutes or look for them on the menu.

He would try to get at least seven hours of sleep a night since sleep is necessary for repair, restoration, and regulation. Sleep plays an important role in stress and appetite. Insufficient amounts of sleep increased the likelihood of obesity. Additionally, sleep deprivation affects the stress hormone cortisol.[131] Steve planned to avoid caffeine after 1p.m. and to limit or eliminate sugar and alcohol intake for the first few weeks. This would allow him to get a longer, more restful sleep.

## Going forward (weight maintenance)

Weight loss is often viewed as a mountain to climb. Once the peak is reached, the quest is over. The person relaxes and reverts to old habits that lead to weight gain. It is very common to see people gain more weight than they lose. Obviously, this is very frustrating. It is easy to see why people give up and resign themselves to being overweight. Steve may occasionally fall back on old habits. He will succeed if the changes he makes turn into a new lifestyle and he can view these lapses as a speed bump and not let them become a setback that allows the return of his ways.

Steve has the tools to lead a healthy life. What he does with these tools and how he proceeds is up to him. He writes the rest of the story.

# ENDNOTES

[1] National Health and Nutrition Examination Survey (NHANES)

[2] Overweight is defined as a Body Mass Index (BMI) of greater than 25%, and obesity is defined as a BMI of greater than 30%. BMI is defined as weight (in kilograms) divided by the square in height in meters.

[3] According to NHANES, the percentage of overweight and obese men, ages 20-74, increased from 54.7% in a 1971-74 survey to 73% in the 2005-08 survey. The number of women who were considered overweight or obese increased from 41.1% in the 1971-74 survey to 62.6% in the 2005-08 survey. (See Table 71, page 263)   The percentage of obesity in men increased from 12.2% to 33.3%, and it increased in women from 16.8% to 36.2%. (See Table 71, page 264). Obesity in children ages 2-5 has gone from 7.2% in the 1988-1994 survey, when they started doing surveys for that age group, to 10.7% in the 2005-08 survey. The percentage of obese children, ages 6 to 11 years, more than quadrupled, increasing from 4.0% in 1971-74 to 17.4% in 2005-08. Obesity in kids age 12 to 19 almost tripled from 6.1% in the early 1970s to 17.9% in 2005-08. (See Table 72, page 267).

[4] Ricardo Uauy and Erik Diaz, *Consequences of food energy excess and positive energy balance*, Public Health Nutrition 8(7A), 1077-1099.

[5] Marja Pyorala, Heikki Miettinen, et al, *Insulin Resistance Syndrome Predicts the Risk of Coronary Heart Disease and Stroke in Healthy Middle-Aged Men: The 22-Year Follow-Up Results of the Helsinki Police Project*, Arterioscle Thromb Vasc Biol 2000;20;538-544.

[6] If you don't produce enough insulin, called type I diabetes, glucose has a difficult time finding its way into your cells. Type I diabetics closely monitor their blood sugar levels and what they eat, and they often take insulin shots.

[7] Additionally, nonalcoholic fatty liver disease is a condition of fat infiltration in the liver and the liver's sign of insulin resistance. Seventy percent of obese persons have nonalcoholic fatty liver disease. This disease can progress to a type of cirrhosis where a liver transplant may be needed.
Mikea C. Devries, Imtiaz A. Samjoo, *Effect of Endurance Exercise on Hepatic Lipid Content, Enzymes and Adiposity in Men and Women,* Obesity Vol. 16 No. 10 Oct. 2008

[8] Blood pressure, historically measured with a blood pressure cuff (sphygmomanometer), is a measure of the pressure when the blood leaves the heart, called systolic pressure, and when the blood enters the heart, called diastolic pressure. The upper number is systolic pressure, and the second smaller number is diastolic pressure.

[9] Packard CJ *Small dense low-density lipoprotein and its role as an independent predictor of cardiovascular disease*, Curr Opin Lipidol. 2006 Aug;17(4):412.

[10] A triglyceride consists of three molecules of fatty acid combined with a molecule of the alcohol glycerol. Triglycerides serve as the backbone of many types of lipids (fats). They are either produced through the digestion of our food or directly by our body.

[11] Rosario Monteiro and Isabel Azevedo, *Chronic Inflammation in Obesity and the Metabolic Syndrome*, Mediators Inflamm. 2010; 2010: 289645. Epub 2010 Jul 14.

[12] BMI is calculated by dividing a person's weight in kilograms by their height in meters squared. If you do not know your BMI and want to know, search the Internet for a BMI calculator. It will ask you your weight and height and magically tell you your BMI.

[13] The most common method for estimating body fat percentage is skinfold calipers. Calipers are used to measure the skinfolds on various parts of your body. Those measurements are used to determine your body fat percentage. This is not a precise measurement, but it can be useful as a means of testing progress if done the same way each time.

It is true that muscle weighs more than fat. Fat mass equals .9 grams per cubic centimeter, and fat-free mass weighs 1.1 grams per cubic centimeter. Hydrostatic Weighing (Hydrodensitometry) uses the principle that fat weighs less than fat-free mass to determine your body fat percentage. You are weighed on land and then asked to strip down to a bathing suit, get into water, exhale, and sink onto a scale. Since fat mass takes up more volume than fat-free mass, you can calibrate body fat percentage using displacement and weight.

The other two tools used to measure body fat are Biomedical Impedance Analysis and Dual Energy X-Ray Absorptiometry (DEXA). Biomedical Impedance Analysis measures your body fat by running an electrical current from either one foot to the other or an arm to a foot. It then calibrates the impedance by using the theory that lean body mass, which contains water, is a good conductor, and body fat, which doesn't contain water, is a poor conductor. Finally, (DEXA) uses X-ray beams to measure bone density, lean body mass, and fat mass. It is considered the gold standard of body mass analysis.

[14] CDC/NCHS, National Health and Nutrition Examination Survey (Table 69, page 256).

[15] U.S. Census Bureau, Statistical Abstract of the United States: 1970 (page 314)

[16] U.S. Census Bureau, Statistical Abstract of the United States: 2011 (page 442)

[17] U.S. Census Bureau, Statistical Abstract of the United States: 1970 (page 218)

[18] U.S. Census Bureau, Statistical Abstract of the United States: 2011 (page 399)

[19] James A. Levine, Norman L. Eberhart, Mike D. Jensen, *Role of Nonexercise Activity Thermogenesis in Resistance to Fat Gain in Humans*, Science Magazine January 8, 1999, Volume 283.

[20] Ibid page 213

[21] James A. Levine, Norman L. Eberhart, Mike D. Jensen, *Role of Nonexercise Activity Thermogenesis in Resistance to Fat Gain in Humans*, Science Magazine January 8, 1999, Volume 283.

[22] James A. Levine, Mark W. Vander Weg, et al., *Non-Exercise Activity Thermogenesis: The Crouching Tiger Hidden Dragon of Societal Weight Gain,* Science Magazine January 2006.

[23] Ibid

[24] James A. Levine, Lorraine M. Lanningham-Foster, et al., *Interindividual Variation in Posture Allocation: Possible Role in Human Obesity,* Science Magazine, January 28, 2005, Vol 307).

[25] Among the current surgical options are gastric bypass surgery and gastric banding surgery. Bypass surgery uses staples or a band to shrink the stomach and limit food intake and nutrient absorption. Gastric banding places a band around the stomach that limits the amount of food you can eat and increases the amount of time the food remains in the stomach.

[26] Dale S. Bond, Suzanne Phelan, et al., *Weight loss maintenance in successful weight losers: surgical versus non-surgical methods,* Int J Obes (Lond), 2009 January; 33(1): 173-180. Doi:10.1038/ijo.2008.256.

[27] Teixeira PJ, Silva MN et al., *Mediators of weight loss and weight loss maintenance in middle-aged women,* Obesity (Silver Spring). 2010 Apr;18(4):725-35. Epub 2009 Aug 20.

[28] In one study, testosterone supplementation increased bone mineral density and reduced stomach fat and total body fat. Enrique Ginzburg, Alvin Lin, et al., *Testosterone and growth hormone normalization: a retrospective study of health outcomes,* Journal of Multidisciplinary Healthcare 2008:1.

[29] Giovanni Corona, MD, Matteo Monami, et al., *Testosterone and Metabolic Syndrome: A Meta-Analysis Study,* J Sex Med 2011;8:272-283.

[30] The prevalence of food allergies and food intolerance is widely debated. If asked, about one in four people thinks they have a food allergy. It turns out the actual number of people with food allergies is much lower. The confirmed diagnosis of food allergies is approximately two to four percent in adults and six to eight percent in children. However, about fifteen to twenty percent of the population has some sort of food intolerance.

Yurdagül Zopf, Dr., Eckhart G. Hahn, Prof. Dr, et. al., *The Differential Diagnosis of Food Intolerance,* Dtsch Arztebl Int. 2009 May; 106(21): 359–370.

[31] Food allergies belong in three categories: IgE mediated allergy, immune cell mediated allergy, or a combination of the two.

Antonella Cianferoni and Jonathan M Spergel, *Food Allergy: Review, Classification and Diagnosis,* Allergology International Vol 58, No4, 2009 457-466.

[32]IgE mediated allergies occur when an antigen found in food binds to the IgE antibody, setting off the immune system response. Watery eyes and runny nose are caused by a chemical called histamines. The IgE mediated allergic response is also responsible for the severe allergic anaphylaxis reaction where the breathing passageways are inhibited. Diagnosis is normally done with a blood or skin prick test, but the accuracy of these tests is questionable. Cell mediated allergies are typically due to a chronic or acute reaction in the gastrointestinal tract. There are few tests that accurately predict cell mediated allergies.

Antonella Cianferoni and Jonathan M Spergel, *Food Allergy: Review, Classification and Diagnosis,*

Allergology International Vol 58, No4, 2009 457-466.

[33] Yurdagül Zopf, Dr., Eckhart G. Hahn, Prof. Dr, et. al., *The Differential Diagnosis of Food Intolerance*, Dtsch Arztebl Int. 2009 May; 106(21): 359–370.

[34] Other forms of food intolerance are histamine and salicylate intolerances. Symptoms of histamine intolerance include flushed skin, itching, congestion, and gastrointestinal issues. Foods high in histamine include long-ripened cheese, red wine, tuna fish, mackerel, and sausage. Symptoms of salicylate intolerance include congestion and gastrointestinal issues. Foods with salicylate content include curry, peppers, oregano, mustard, and cayenne pepper.

Yurdagül Zopf, Dr., Eckhart G. Hahn, Prof. Dr, et. al., *The Differential Diagnosis of Food Intolerance*, Dtsch Arztebl Int. 2009 May; 106(21): 359–370.

[35] P.R. Shewry, *Wheat*, Journal of Experimental Botany, (209) Vol. 60, No. 6, pp 1537-1553.

[36] Gluten is a combination of prolamin, which is primarily gliadin, and glutenin found in wheat, rye, and barley.

[37] Celiac disease is an inflammatory condition of the small intestine triggered by the consumption of gluten. Celiac disease takes away the villi in the small intestine. It affects approximately two to three million people but only 15% to 20% of those who have it have been diagnosed with it.

[38] Lieberman, Shari, *The Gluten Connection: how gluten sensitivity may be sabotaging your weight and your health – what you can do to take control now* (2007).

[39] A study of 183 healthy females ages ranging from 18 to 81 were tested and it was determined that their resting metabolic rate was not age related but corresponded with their fat free mass.

Eric T. Poehlman, Mike I. Goran, et al., *Determinants of decline in resting metabolic rate in aging in females*, AJP-Endo March 1993 Vol. 264 No. 3 E450-E455

[40] Hormonal changes, a decrease in muscle protein synthesis, oxidative stress, and inactivity contribute to the loss of muscle.

[41] T. Lang, T. Streeper, P. Cawthon, et al., *Sarcopenia: etiology, clinical consequences, intervention, and assessment*, Osteoporos Int (2010) 21:543-559 page 551.

[42] Interval training or some other form of strenuous activity recruits type II muscle fibers and increases their mitochondrial content.

John O. Holloszy and Edward F. Coyle, *Adaptations of skeletal muscle in endurance exercise and their metabolic consequences*, J. Appl. Physiol.: Respirat. Environ.Physiol. (1984) 56(4): 831-838, page 833.

[43] In one study, men were able to increase their basal metabolic rate by over five percent with just ten weeks of resistance training or a combination of resistance training and endurance training.

*Concurrent resistance and endurance training influence basal metabolic rate in nondieting individuals.* by Brett A. Dolezal and Jeffrey A. Potteiger J. Appl Physiol 85:695-700, 1998.

[44] Under certain conditions, resistance training has a positive impact on calories expended well after

working out. During resistance training we are breaking down muscles. The process of rebuilding them requires energy and is defined as excess post-exercise oxygen consumption or EPOC. The number of calories used to rebuild muscles after exercise appears to depend on the intensity of the training, but studies have shown a twenty percent increase in metabolism over a 48-hour period in young men participating in just three weight lifting exercises of high intensity.

Mark D. Schuenke, Richard P. Milak and Jeffrey M. McBride, *Effect of an acute period resistance exercise on excess post-exercise oxygen consumption: implications for body mass management*, Eur J Appl Physiol (2002) 86: 411-417.

[45] I.G. Fatouros, S. Tournis, D. Leontsini et al., *Leptin and Adiponectin Responses in Overweight Inactive Elderly Following Resistance Training and Detraining Are Intensity Related*, The J. Clin. Endocrinol. 2005 90:5970-5977, Table 2.

[46] Resistance exercise has also been shown to have a positive effect on anabolic hormones, growth hormones, cortisol, and chronic insulin-like growth factors adaption with resistance training.

William J. Kraemer and Nicholas A. Ratamess, *Hormonal Response and Adaptations to Resistance Exercise and Training*, Sport Med 2005 35(4) 339-361, page 341-42.

[47] The technical definition of a calorie is the amount of energy it takes to heat one gram of water one degree Celsius. A food calorie is really 1,000 calories or a kcal. But for our purposes when we refer to the calorie we are referring to kcals or food calories. If you wanted to calculate the exact amount of calories a food contained, you could go to a lab and burn the food in a bomb calorimeter and see how many degrees a given amount of water rises. However, the calories of most foods are measured indirectly using The Atwater System. The Atwater System measures the grams of proteins, fats, and carbohydrates (together called macronutrients) in the food.

[48] Normally, insoluble fiber is subtracted from the carbohydrate count before calculating calories from carbohydrates.

[49] In a long-term study, researchers assessed the changes in waist circumference and body mass index and how they related to food intake in a group of men and women. They measured the participants at a baseline and 5-1/2 years later. The authors concluded that diets consisting of high-energy-density foods were strong predictors of a gain in visceral fat.

Romaguera D, Angquist L, Du H, Jakobsen MU, Forouhi NG, et al. (2010) *Dietary Determinants of Changes in Waist Circumstance Adjusted for Body Mass Index – a Proxy Measure of Visceral Adiposity*. PLoS ONE 5(7): e11588. Doi10.1371/Journal.pone0011588.

[50] Lipolysis, the breakdown of triglycerides into glycerol and fatty free acids, and gluconeogenesis, the process where fat is used as energy, are suppressed because this new food will take the place of these fats. Among the problems with insulin resistance is that lypolysis is inhibited, and therefore triglycerides continue to break down while new ones are being ingested.

William E. Kraus and Cris A. Slentz, *Exercise Training, Lipid Regulation, and Insulin Action: A Tangled Web of Cause and Effect*, Obesity December 2009 Vol. 17 Supplement 3 S21-S26.

[51] Carbohydrate digestion starts in the mouth and in the stomach until the acids in the stomach stop the

digestion. Carbohydrates then enter the small intestine where, with help from the pancreas, they are broken down further into glucose. Glucose then enters the bloodstream. In response to the glucose entering the bloodstream, the pancreas secretes insulin.

[52] HFCS 55 is a combination of 55% fructose and about 45% glucose. It can be found in many soft drinks. HFCS 42 is a combination of 42% fructose and 55% glucose and is found in food. Table sugar, by comparison, is 50% fructose and 50% glucose.

[53] Salwa W. Rizkalla, *Health implications of fructose consumption: A review of recent data*, Nutrition & Metabolism 2010 7:82.

[54] Mark J. Dekker, Qiaozhu Su et al., *Fructose: a highly lipogenic nutrient implicated in insulin resistance, hepatic steatosis, and the metabolic syndrome*, AM J Physiol Endocrinol Metab 299:E685-E694, 2010.

[55] In a recent study, obese or overweight men and women in their mid-fifties ingested twenty-five percent of their calorie intake as either glucose or fructose over a two-week period. Both groups increased weight, body fat, and waist circumference. However, the fructose-fed participants showed a much greater increase in visceral fat, greater hepatic de novo lipogenesis (the process of turning carbohydrate into fat in the liver), an increase in small dense LDL concentrations (associated with atherogenesis or plaque growing in the arteries), and decreased insulin sensitivity.

Fructose does not require insulin for the initial steps of its liver metabolism, which means it is digested without the normal sugar-regulating hormone. Fructose also promotes lipogenesis, the process where sugars are converted into fats.

Stanhope, KL, Schwarz JM, Keim NL, et al., *Consuming fructose-sweetened, not glucose-sweetened, beverages increases visceral adiposity and lipids and decreases insulin sensitivity in overweight/obese humans*, J Clin Invest 119: 1322-1334, 2009.

[56] Dietary fiber is either soluble—fiber that is fermented in the colon—or insoluble fiber, which is fiber with bulking action but only slightly fermented in the colon. The main source of insoluble fiber is corn, wheat, and bran. The main source of soluble fiber is fruits and vegetables. Oat and barley contain both insoluble and soluble fiber.

Paresh Dandona, Husam Ghanim et al., *Macronutrient intake induces oxidative and inflammatory stress: potential relevance to atherosclerosis and insulin resistance,* Experimental and Molecular Medicine, Vol. 4, 245-253, April 2010.

[57] Martin O. Weickert and Andreas F. H. Pfeiffer, *Metabolic Effects of Dietary Fiber Consumption and Prevention of Diabetes, J. Nutr. March 1, 2008* vol. 138, no. 3 439-442.

[58] *In 1981, a group from the University of Toronto developed the glycemic index. The researchers fed subjects varying foods containing 50 grams of carbohydrates and then measured their glucose response. They compared the response time to the response if they were fed 50 grams of straight glucose. Glucose has an index of 100. The index of other foods is calculated as a percentage of glucose.*

*David J.A. Jenkins, D.M., Thomas M.S. Woever, et al., Glycemic index of foods: a physiological basis for carbohydrate exchange, Am J Clin Nutr March 1981* vol. 34 no. 3 362-366.

[59] Simin Liu, JoAnn E Manson, et al., *Dietary glycemic load assessed by food-frequency questionnaire in relation to plasma high-density-lipoprotein cholesterol and fasting plasma triacylglycerols in postmenopausal women, Am J Clin Nutr March 2001* vol. 73 no. 3 560-566.

[60] Mulkamal, K.J., Kuller, L.H., *et al. Prospective study of alcohol consumption and risk of dementia in older adults. Journal of the American Medical Association*, 2003 (March 19), *289*, 1405-1413.

[61] Alcohol is broken down in the liver and is initially converted to a highly reactive and toxic molecule, acetaldehyde. With moderate consumption, alcohol is converted from that molecule to acetate. Higher alcohol consumption leads to an increase in highly reactive oxygen radicals. Oxygen radicals play a role in a number of health issues.

Charles S. Lieber, Pathways of Alcohol Metabolism, Alcohol Research & Health Vol. 27, No. 3, 2003, 225.

[62] Charles S. Lieber, M.D.,M.A.C.P., Relationships Between Nutrition, Alcohol Use, and Liver Disease, Alcohol Research & Health Vol. 27, No. 3, 2003 220-231.

[63] People tend to overestimate their energy expenditure when exercising by three or four times. And when asked to eat in calories what they burned exercising, they eat two to three times more than they burned.

Willbond SM, Laviolette MA, Duval K, Doucet E., *Normal weight men and women overestimate exercise energy expenditure,* J Sports Med Phys Fitness. 2010 Dec; 50(4):377-84.

[64] Warbuton, DER, Nicol C, Bredin SS (2006a). *Health benefits of physical activity: the evidence.* Can Med Assoc J, 174, 801-809.

[65] Researchers investigated the effect exercise and diet had on adiponectin over a 12-week period. Adiponectin is a protein secreted in fat tissue that helps regulate insulin sensitivity and reduce inflammation. Normally, adiponectin amounts are lower in obese individuals. With exercise and diet, obese people can increase adiponectin amounts by as much as 20 percent over a short period of time.

Tore Christiansen, Soren K. Paulsen, et al., *Diet-Induced Weight Loss and Exercise Alone and in Combination Enhance the Expression of Adiponectin Receptors in Adipose Tissue and Skeletal Muscle, but Only Diet-Induced Weight Loss Enhanced Circulating Adiponectin*, J Clin Endorcrinol Metab, February 2010, 95(2):911-919

[66] Joanna Kruck, *Physical Activity and Health*, Asian Pacific J Cancer Prev, 10, 721-728.

[67] In 1995, the Center for Disease Control and the American College of Sports Medicine issued their recommendations for leisure time exercise activity. In 2005, they reviewed the results. Over 23% of adults reported that they were physically inactive. Almost half of the adults reported that they had not met the minimum activity recommended by the 1995 report. In 2005, the American College of Sports Medicine, with an endorsement from the American Heart Association, revised their recommendations based on new research. The recommendations were for adults age 18 to 65.

The panel recommends a minimum of 30 minutes of moderate-intensity aerobic activity 5 days a week or vigorous activity 20 minutes a day three days a week. They also recommend resistance training a minimum of two non-consecutive days a week. The resistance training should consist of 8 to 10 exercises emphasizing the major muscle groups. Each exercise should include 8 to 12 repetitions done to "volitional fatigue."

Haskell WL, LEE, I, Pate RR, et al., *Physical Activity and Public Health: Updated Recommendation for Adults from the American College of Sports Medicine and the American Heart Association*, Med Sci Sports Exerc. 2007 Aug;39(8):1423-34.

[68] Jurca, R., M. J. Lamonte, T. S. Church, et al., *Associations of Muscle Strength and Aerobic Fitness with Metabolic Syndrome in Men.* Med. Sci.Sports Exerc., Vol. 36, No. 8, pp. 1301–1307, 2004.

[69] Brian D. Duscha, Cris A. Slentz et al., *Effects of exercise training amount and intensity on peak oxygen consumption in middle-age men and women at risk for cardiovascular disease*, Chest. 2005 Oct;128(4):2788-93.

[70] Additionally, aerobic capacity has proven to be a more powerful predictor of survival than other risk factors among healthy men and men with cardiovascular disease.

D. Ennette Larson-Meyer, Leanne Redman, et al., *Caloric Restriction with or without Exercise: The Fitness vs. Fatness Debate*, Med Sci Sports Exerc. 2010 January; 42(1): 152-159.

[71] A trained endurance athlete uses less carbohydrates and more fat oxidation during submaximal performance. *Adaptations of skeletal muscle in endurance exercise and their metabolic consequences* by John O. Holloszy and Edward F. Coyle J. Appl. Physiol.: Respirat. Environ.Physiol. 56(4): 831-838, 1984.

[72] Researchers tested seven healthy untrained males after five and 31 days of prolonged endurance exercise. The participants' fat oxidation (fat loss while sitting around) increased by approximately eleven percent.

S.M. Phillips, H.J. Green et al., *Effects of training duration on substrate turnover and oxidation during exercise, Journal of Applied Physiology November 1996 vol. 81 no. 5* 2182-2191.

[73] They also concluded that cardio-respiratory fitness may have contributed to cholesterol changes independent of weight loss.

K.R. Wilund, L.A. Feeney, et at., Effects of Endurance Exercise Training on Markers of Cholesterol Absorption and Synthesis, Physiol Res 58: 545-552 (2009).

[74] Stephen H. Boutcher, *High-Intensity Intermittent Exercise and Fat Loss*, Journal of Obesity Volume 2011 10 pages

[75] The participants also increased their oxygen intake capacity. The studies were conducted over periods ranging from six weeks to twenty-four weeks.

Stephen H. Boutcher, *High-Intensity Intermittent Exercise and Fat Loss*, Journal of Obesity Volume 2011 10 pages

[76] Z. Zadak, R. Hyspler, et al., *Antioxidants and Vitamins in Clinical Conditions*, Physiol. Res. 58 (Suppl. 1): S13-S17, 2009.

[77] Earl S. Ford, Ali H. Mokdad, et al., *The Metabolic Syndrome and Antioxidant Concentrations; Findings From the Third National Health and Nutrition Examination Survey*, Diabetes, Vol. 52, Sept 2003.

[78] Richard D. Semba, Fulvio Lauretani, and Luigi Ferrucci, *Carotenoids as protection against sarcopenia in*

*older adults*, Arch Biochem Biophys. 2007 February 15; 458(2): 141–145.

[79] DL Waters, RN Baumgartner, PJ Garry, and B Vellas, *Advantages of dietary, exercise-related, and therapeutic interventions to prevent and treat sarcopenia in adult patients: an update*, Clinical Interventions in Aging 2010:5 259-270.

[80] In a study of women participating in the Nurses' Health Study, researchers compared diets with higher intakes of vegetables, fruits, legumes (such as peas and beans), whole grains, fish, and poultry to diets with higher intakes of red meat, processed meat, refined grains, sweets, desserts, french fries, and high-fat dairy products. The diet with more red and processed meats had higher markers for inflammation, including C-reactive protein, which has been shown to play a role in plaque buildup in blood vessels.

Esther Lopez-Garcia, Matthias B Schulze, et al., *Major dietary patterns are related to plasma concentrations of markers of inflammation and endothelial dysfunction*, Am J Clin Nutr October 2004 vol. 80 no. 4 *1029-1035.*

[81] In another study, researchers fed overweight men an anti-inflammatory dietary mix of fish oil, green tea extract, vitamin E, vitamin C, tomato extract and resveratol. Markers for inflammation and oxidative stress both declined after five weeks on the diet. Specifically, inflammatory receptors associated with fat tissues were reduced, plasma triglycerides were reduced, and markers indicating endothelial, or blood vessel function, were increased.

Gertruud CM Bakker,Marjan J van Erk, *An antiinflammatory dietary mix modulates inflammation and oxidative and metabolic stress in overweight men: a nutrigenomics approach*, Am J Clin Nutr April 2010 vol. 91 no. 4 1044-1059.

[82] Paresh Dandona, Husam Ghanim et al., *Macronutrient intake induces oxidative and inflammatory stress: potential relevance to atherosclerosis and insulin resistance*, Experimental and Molecular Medicine, Vol. 4, 245-253, April 2010.

[83] Flavenoids are also known as flavonols, flavones, isoflavones, tannins, and catechins.

[84] Researchers investigated the role of flavenoids in obesity in a large group of Netherlands women over a fourteen-year period. Women with higher flavonoid intake had significantly lower BMI increases than the general group. They found the flavenoid with the greatest association to lower BMI increases came from a flavanol called myricetin, found in teas, leeks, and onions.

Laura AE Hughes, Ilja CW Arts, et al., *Higher dietary flavones, flavonol, and certain catechin intakes are associated with less of an increase in BMI over time in women: a longitudinal analysis from the Netherlands Cohort Study*, Am J Clin Nut 2008;88:1341-52.

[85] Gary R. Beecher, Overview of *Dietary Flavonoids: Nomenclature, Occurrence and Intake*, J. Nutr. 133: 3248S-3254S, 2003.

[86] DL Waters, RN Baumgartner, PJ Garry, and B Vellas, *Advantages of dietary, exercise-related, and therapeutic interventions to prevent and treat sarcopenia in adult patients: an update*, Clinical Interventions in Aging 2010:5 259-270.

[87] Paresh Dandona, Husam Ghanim et al., *Macronutrient intake induces oxidative and inflammatory stress:*

*potential relevance to atherosclerosis and insulin resistance,* Experimental and Molecular Medicine, Vol. 4, 245-253, April 2010.

[88] Coenzyme $Q_{10}$ is a substance generated by the body and found in certain foods that plays a critical role in the generation of energy in the body. It also acts as an antioxidant. It sits in the mitochondria, where it plays its energy production role, or it circulates in the bloodstream. It circulates in the bloodstream in fat cells and thus is directly correlated with blood levels of cholesterol.

Sarah L Molyneux, Joanna M Young, et al., *Coenzyme Q10: Is There a Clinical Role and a Case for Measurement?,* Clin Biochem Rev Vol 29 May 2008 71-82.

[89] In one study, physical inactivity correlated with elevated levels of white blood cells. The white blood cells were reduced after 12 weeks of exercise three days a week.

Kyle L. Timmerman, Mike G. Flynn et at., *Exercise training-induced lowering of inflammatory (CD14+CD16+) monocytes: a role in the anti-inflammatory influence of exercise?,* Journal of Leukocyte Biology Vol. 84, Nov 2008.

[90] They are the primary source of blood cells, muscle, bone, hormones, and enzymes that catalyze metabolic reactions and signal intermediaries between and within cells.

Zhenqi Liu and Eugene J. Barrett, *Human protein metabolism: its measurement and* regulation, Am J Physiol Endocrinol Metab 283: E1105-E1112, 2002 10.1152/ajpendo.00337.2002.

[91] Dietary proteins are broken down into polypeptides (strings of amino acids), starting in the stomach by pepsin. The polypeptides are further broken down into small peptides or individual amino acids in the small intestine. They end up in the liver, where they are either synthesized into new amino acids or sent off into the bloodstream to perform other tasks such as forming hemoglobin (which transports oxygen throughout the body), hormones, enzymes, and antibodies.

[92] Our bodies require twice as much energy to synthesize proteins as it does to store either carbohydrates or fat. Thus, the turnover of protein from breakdown to build-up requires at least five percent of our resting energy expenditure.

Zhenqi Liu and Eugene J. Barrett, *Human protein metabolism: its measurement and regulation,* Am J Physiol Endocrinol Metab 283: E1105-E1112, 2002 10.1152/ajpendo.00337.2002.

[93] The nine essential amino acids are: leucine, isoleucine, lysine, threonine, valine, phenylalanine, tryptophan, methionine, and histidine.

[94] Joint FAO/WHO/UNU Expert Consultation on Protein and Amino Acid Requirements in Human Nutrition (2002 : Geneva, Switzerland).

[95] In a paper reviewing the research on the relationship between protein intake and renal or kidney disease, the authors found that excess protein increases calcium and uric acid but did not find evidence of kidney disease even in athletes who ingested over 2 grams of protein per kilogram of weight.

William F Martin, Lawrence E. Armstrong and Nancy R Rodriquez, *Dietary protein intake and renal function,* Nutrition & Metabolism 2005, 2:25 doi:10.1186/1743-7075-2-25.

[96] It may also aid in reducing fat accumulation and plasma lipids in adipose and liver tissue. This in turn could reduce the risk of several obesity issues including atherosclerosis.

Manuel T. Velasquez and Sam J. Bhathena, *Role of Dietary Soy Protein in Obesity*, Int. J. Med. Sci., 4(2):72-82 9.

[97] G. Harvey Anderson and Shannon E. Moore, *Dietary Proteins in the Regulation of Food Intake and Body Weight in Humans*, J. Nutr. April 1, 2004 vol. 134 no. 4 974S-979S.

[98] Fatty acids are stored in adipocytes (fat tissue) as triglycerol and in our muscles as triglycerides. Fat tissue is found mostly in the abdominal cavity and in subcutaneous tissue. Triglycerides stored in the muscle provide a large source of energy. In addition to energy use, fats act as insulation for our vital organs and our body to outside heat. They are used to store fat-soluble vitamins such as A, D, E, and K.

[99] Saturated fats are fats with the maximum number of hydrogen atoms attached to each carbon atom. The main types of saturated fats found in human foods are palmitic acid, stearic acid, and lauric acid. Foods with palimitc acid include dairy and beef. Foods with stearic acid include cocoa butter and animal and plant fats. Foods with lauric acid include palm kernel oil, milk, and coconut oil.

[100] Patty W Siri-Tarino, Qi Sun, et al., *Saturated fat, carbohydrate and cardiovascular disease*, AM J Clin Nutr 2010;91:502-9

[101] *Myriam A.M.A. Thijssen, Gerard Hornstra, and Ronald P. Mensink, Stearic, Oleic, and Linoleic Acids Have Comparable Effects on Markers of Thrombotic Tendency in Health Human Subjects, J. Nutr.* December 1, 2005 vol. 135 no. 12 2805-2811.

[102] Monounsaturated fats are fatty acids that are missing one pair of hydrogen atoms. The two main monounsaturated fats found in the diet are palmitoleic acid and oleic acid. Oleic acid is the main source of monounsaturated fats found in foods. It is found in avocado, olive oil, canola oil, and grapeseed oil. Palmitoleic acid is found in macadamia nuts, some fish oils, and beef fat.

[103] Ancel Keys, Alessandro Menotti, et al., *The Diet And 15-Year Death Rate In The Seven Countries Study*, Am. J. Epidemiol. (1986) 124 (6):903-915.

[104] Nimer Assy, Faris Nassar, et. al, *Olive oil consumption and non-alcoholic fatty liver disease*, World J Gastroenterol 2009 April 21; 15(15): 1809-1815.

[105] In an effort to make unsaturated fat oils more solid, a process called hydrogenation is used. In this process, hydrogen molecules are added to the oil, and the fat is turned into a semi-solid saturated fat.

[106] Trans-fatty acids are unsaturated fats where the carbon-to-carbon double bonds sit opposite one another on the molecule.

Lenore Arab, *Biomarkers of Fat and Fatty Acid Intake*, J. Nutr. March 1, 2003, vol. 133 no. 3 925S-932S, page 927S.

[107] Omega-6 fatty acids (linoleic acid and arachidonic acid) are stored in cell membranes and can be mobilized by phospholipids. They are the principle precursor in eicosanoids, which are local hormones that have a number of roles in the body, including the reducing inflammation, regulating blood pressure

and body temperature,, and promoting tissue growth. There are a number of Omega-6 fatty acids, but linoleic acid is a key source of polyunsaturated fats in the diet.

Lenore Arab, *Biomarkers of Fat and Fatty Acid Intake, J. Nutr.* March 1, 2003 vol. 133 no. 3 925S-932S.

[108] Omega-3 fatty acids also play an important role in eicosanoid production and, therefore, compete with Omega-6 fatty acids. Where Omega-6 fatty acids are pro-inflammatory, Omega-3 fatty acids play an anti-inflammatory role.

[109] Olivier Molendi-Coste, Vanessa Legry, and Isabelle A. Leclercq, *"Why and How to Meet n-3 PUFA Dietary Recommendations?"* Gastroenterology Research and Practice, vol. 2011, Article ID 364040, 11 pages, 2011. doi:10.1155/2011/364040.

[110] Paresh Dandona, Husam Ghanim et al., *Macronutrient intake induces oxidative and inflammatory stress: potential relevance to atherosclerosis and insulin resistance,* Experimental and Molecular Medicine, Vol. 4, 245-253, April 2010.

[111] In an article reviewing the effects of ALA, the type of Omega-3 fatty acid found in flaxseed oil, the reviewers did not find protective associations between it and heart failure. Fish contains EPA and DHA, the fatty acids found to be the most beneficial to our health.

Johanna M. Geleijnse & Janette de Goede & Ingeborg A. Brouwer, *Alpha-Linolenic Acid: Is It Essential to Cardiovascular Health?,* Curr Atheroscler Rep (2010) 12:359–36.

[112] Japan and Iceland, two countries with the highest ratio of Omega-3 to Omega-6 fatty acids, also have the lowest mortality rates from cardiovascular disease, coronary heart disease, and strokes. Japan also has a very low percentage of major depression in their population. The ratio of Omega-3 fatty acids to Omega-6 fatty acids in those countries is six Omega-3 acids to four Omega-6.

Joseph R Hibbeln, Levi RG Nieminen, et al., *Healthy intakes of n-3 and n-6 fatty acids: estimations considering worldwide diversity,* Am J Clin 2006;83 (suppl):1483S-93S.

[113] In a recent study, symptoms of depression were lower in persons with high levels of Omega-3 fatty acids and higher in persons with high levels of the Omega-6 fatty acid. Additionally, a high ratio of Omega-6 fatty acids to Omega-3 fatty acids was positively correlated with symptoms of depression.

Sarah M. Conklin, Stephen B. Manuck, et al., High w-6 and Low w-3 Fatty Acids are Associated With Depressive Symptoms and Neuroticism, Psychosomatic Medicine 69:932-934 (2007).

[114] Vitamins are either fat soluble or water soluble. Fat soluble vitamins, vitamins A, D, E, K, are stored in the liver and fat cells. Water soluble vitamins such as vitamin C and the B vitamins are not stored in your body making it more likely to have a deficiency if not ingested or taken in a supplement.

[115] Susan Cheng, Joseph M. Massaro, Caroline S. Fox, et al., *Adiposity, Cardiometabolic Risk, and Vitamin D Status: The Framington Heart Study,* Diabetes, Vol. 59, 242-248 (2010).

[116] Vitamin D deficiency has also been linked to osteomalacia (a softening of the bones), cancer, autoimmune disease, and infection. In children, severe vitamin D deficiency can cause rickets, which causes bones to fail to mineralize, resulting in delayed development, failure to thrive, and skeletal abnormalities.

William G. Tsiaras and Martin A. Weinstock, *Factors Influencing Vitamin D Status*, Acta Derm Veverol 2011; 91: 115-124.

[117] William G. Tsiaras and Martin A. Weinstock, *Factors Influencing Vitamin D Status*, Acta Derm Veverol 2011; 91: 115-124.

[118] Deficiencies of vitamin $B_{12}$ generally come from the inability to absorb it. A deficiency can cause neurological damage as well as fatigue, weakness, and loss of appetite.

[119] It also aids in producing certain hormones in the adrenal gland. High doses, under medical supervision, have been used to lower LDL cholesterol and triglycerides.

[120] With vitamins $B_6$ and $B_{12}$, it lowers blood homocysteine levels. (Homocysteine is an amino acid that may promote atherosclerosis or the thickening of blood vessels.) Women who want to get pregnant should consult with their physician because they may need folic acid supplementation.

[121] Choline is also essential to the synthesis of phosolipids in cell membranes.

[122] Laura M. Plum, Lothar Rink, and Hajo Haase, *The Essential Toxin: Impact of Zinc on Human Health*, Int J Environ Res Public Health. 2010 April; 7(4): 1342–1365.

[123] David O. Kennedy, Rachel Veasey, et al., *Effects of high-dose B vitamin complex with vitamin C and minerals on subjective mood and performance in healthy males,* Psychopharmacology (Berl). 2010 July; 211(1): 55–68.

[124] Robert M. Sapolsky, <u>Why Zebras Don't Get Ulcers</u> (1994, Holt/Owl 3rd Rep. Ed. 2004).

[125] Mary F. Dallman, *Stress-induced obesity and the emotional nervous system*, Trends Endocrinol Metab. 2010 March; 21(3): 159-165.

[126] Rena R Wing and Suzanne Phelan, *Long-Term weight loss maintenance*, Am J Clin Nutr 2005;82 (suppl):222S-5S.

[127] Davis LM, Coleman C, et al., *Efficacy of a meal replacement diet plan compared to a food-based diet plan after a period of weight loss and weight maintenance: a randomized controlled trial*, Nutr J. 2010 Mar 11;9:11.

[128] Manzoni GM, Pagnini F, et al., *Internet-based behavioral interventions for obesity: an updated systematic review*, Clin Pract Epidemiol Ment Health. 2011 Mar 4;7:19-28.

[129] Daniel A. Judelson, Carl M. Marsh et al., *Effect of hydration state on resistance exercise-induced endocrine markers of anabolism, catabolism, and metabolism*, J Appl Physiol 105:816-824, 2008.

[130] Ann C. Grandjean and Nicole R. Grandjean, *Dehydration and Cognitive Performance*, Jam Coll Nutr, Vol. 26, No. 5, 549S-554S (2007).

[131] Rachel Leproult and Eve Van Cauter, *Role of Sleep and Sleep Loss in Hormonal Release and Metabolism*, Endocr Dev. 2010 ; 17: 11–21. doi:10.1159/000262524.

# ABOUT THE AUTHOR

## Gregg Ghelfi, NSCA-CPT, JD, LLM

After graduating from the University of Notre Dame law school, Gregg Ghelfi practiced law and ran several businesses. After seeing the consequences of obesity first hand, he founded fitinthemiddle.com, a website dedicated to fitness, nutrition and weight loss. He is a certified personal trainer and First Line Therapy Lifestyle Educator who works with people with Metabolic Syndrome. He has written several articles on health and fitness. He believes that physical and mental fitness through exercise and nutrition are critical to leading happy and productive lives.

## Bob Ghelfi, MD, MBA, FACS

Bob Ghelfi, M.D. owns and operates BodyLogicMD of Sacramento. He is a member of Member of the Fellowship for Anti-Aging and Regenerative and Functional Medicine. He treats men and women for hormonal imbalances using bio-identical hormone therapy. He also works with clients on nutrition and fitness programs. Dr. Ghelfi also practices as a surgeon in Redding California where he is often confronted with the consequences of poor choices. Certified in A4M/Anti-Aging medicine and Board Certified in General Surgery.

## Marilee Tatom, RN, BSN

Marilee has been a registered nurse since 1992. She is certified with the American Academy of Anti-Aging Medicine. She is also a certified operating room nurse. She is an avid runner and a "health nut." She currently works alongside Dr. Bob Ghelfi, medical director of BodyLogicMD of Sacramento, CA as a nurse and office manager. She also works at Mercy Medical Center in Redding, CA as an operating nurse. Certified in A4M/Anti-Aging medicine.

www.ingramcontent.com/pod-product-compliance
Lightning Source LLC
Chambersburg PA
CBHW060907280326
41934CB00007B/1227